A Companion to the Classification of Mental Disorders

A Companion to the Classification of Mental Disorders

John E. Cooper
Emeritus Professor of Psychiatry,
University of Nottingham,
Nottingham, UK

Norman Sartorius
Former Director of Division of Mental Health,
The World Health Organization,
Geneva, Switzerland

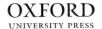
OXFORD
UNIVERSITY PRESS

OXFORD
UNIVERSITY PRESS

Great Clarendon Street, Oxford, OX2 6DP,
United Kingdom

Oxford University Press is a department of the University of Oxford.
It furthers the University's objective of excellence in research, scholarship,
and education by publishing worldwide. Oxford is a registered trade mark of
Oxford University Press in the UK and in certain other countries

Published in the United States of America by Oxford University Press
198 Madison Avenue, New York, NY 10016, United States of America

British Library Cataloguing in Publication Data
Data available

Library of Congress Control Number: 2013941075

ISBN 978–0–19–966949–3

Printed and bound by
CPI Group (UK) Ltd, Croydon, CR0 4YY

Oxford University Press makes no representation, express or implied, that the
drug dosages in this book are correct. Readers must therefore always check
the product information and clinical procedures with the most up-to-date
published product information and data sheets provided by the manufacturers
and the most recent codes of conduct and safety regulations. The authors and
the publishers do not accept responsibility or legal liability for any errors in the
text or for the misuse or misapplication of material in this work. Except where
otherwise stated, drug dosages and recommendations are for the non-pregnant
adult who is not breastfeeding.

Links to third party websites are provided by Oxford in good faith and
for information only. Oxford disclaims any responsibility for the materials
contained in any third party website referenced in this work.

Acknowledgements

We have been fortunate to share some distinguished senior colleagues who provided advice and encouragement on both sides of the Atlantic over the course of many years, particularly Aubrey Lewis, Joseph Zubin, Morton Kramer, Michael Shepherd, and John Wing. Between them they provided the administrative, financial, and background support without which much of what is described in this book would have been truncated or impossible.

On a more contemporary note, it is also a pleasure to acknowledge the shared interest and stimulation derived from working on many of the topics described here with Assen Jablensky, Darrel Regier, Michael Rutter, Gerald Klerman, Leon Eisenberg, Raymond Sadoun, Charles Pull, Aksel Bertelson, Bedirhan Ustun, Sasha Janca, and many others. We also wish to thank Mrs L. Kurk for her excellent help in handling the administrative tasks related to the production of this book.

Contents

Introduction

Contemporary psychiatric classifications such as ICD-10 and DSM-IV do not exist in isolation. They rest upon a firm foundation of several decades of descriptive psychiatry during which the symptoms and syndromes upon which their categories are based have been identified and described reliably in many different cultures. To understand how these classifications have been developed and to appreciate that they have both benefits and limitations, it is necessary to know something about this background. One of the main purposes of this book is to illustrate and comment upon this development process, which has entailed a great deal of international and cross-cultural cooperation. The reader may also be interested by comments upon topics and problems which are not usually found in textbooks or covered in conventional courses on mental health issues.

A variety of psychiatric classifications was developed in many countries before the realization that internationally acceptable methods of description and classification were needed. What might be called 'the modern era' began in the 1950s, and Stengel's review for the World Health Organization (Stengel 1960), has been taken as signalling the start of this. Those readers who are interested in the history of psychiatric classification before this are recommended to start with publications such as *Sources and Traditions of Classification in Psychiatry* (Sartorius, Jablensky, et al. 1990).

The general plan of the book

The book starts with some examples of what can happen in the absence of an internationally agreed psychiatric classification. These examples are placed first as a warning, in the hope that they will awaken some interest even in those who usually regard classification as a tiresome chore. The chapters then move on to describe how classifications that can serve as a common language, such as ICD-10 Chapter V and DSM-IV, were gradually developed. A number of chapters then discuss selected basic issues and problems that are as yet unsolved. These are to do with the process and methods of classification, and not with the detailed content of present or future classifications. The book is laid out in a comparatively large number of short chapters, with liberal use of numbered sections. This should aid the reader when navigating around the chapters in search of particular topics.

In more detail

The order of Chapters 2 to 7 is largely determined by the chronological order of the events and processes by which progress towards international agreement about diagnosis and classification was gradually achieved. Chapter 8 contains a discussion of an important question to which there is as yet no simple answer—'To what extent are complaints as expressed by the subject, equivalent to the symptoms inferred by the psychiatrist?' The problems of translation of interview schedules, their use in different cultures and the search for equivalence of meaning are dealt with in Chapter 9. In Chapter 10 there are comments upon the development of ICD-9 and the achievement of greater agreement between ICD-10 and DSM-IV, by means of some of the activities in the Joint Project between the NIMH and the WHO. The justification for different versions of a classification for different purposes is explained in Chapter 11.

Chapter 12 is a diversion from psychiatry, in that it deals with the general process of classification. It contains a brief account of the useful classifications in biology and the physical sciences, in order to see if any lessons might be learned from them that might be of benefit to psychiatry.

Chapter 13 is devoted to problems that have to be dealt with by compilers of classifications of anything, but which become particularly prominent when attempts are made to develop a classification for use in psychiatry. Concise and useful definitions of disease and psychiatric disorder remain elusive.

Chapter 14 presents some basic problems and processes by which psychiatric diagnoses are made, and goes into the relative merits and drawbacks of using lists of diagnostic criteria and narrative descriptions. The limitations of diagnostic classifications are noted in Chapter 15, together with the classification of disability. Chapter 16 discusses multi-axial classifications; these are needed because of the differences between a classification of diseases, a classification of persons with diseases, and a classification of encounters between mental health professionals. For many psychiatric patients, descriptive classifications of the patient's characteristics, such as disability and relationships with other persons, are just as useful as the diagnosis of the illness, and special arrangements are needed for this. Chapter 17 takes a wider international view of psychiatric classification and, together with Appendix 4, goes into the 'meta effects' of psychiatric classifications, that is, the effects of psychiatric classifications beyond psychiatry itself. Chapter 18 is a brief discussion of how to get the most out of using psychiatric classifications, and how to avoid the pitfalls of using them badly.

Chapter 19 contains only brief notes on the final stages of the development of ICD-11 and DSM-5; this is because at the time of writing the only items of public knowledge about these complicated processes are the proposed timetables for publication. It finishes with some speculations on the more remote future of psychiatric classifications.

Some underlying issues

Many of the problems discussed in this book stem from the fact that psychiatric diagnoses are often not of the same nature as the diagnoses made in other branches of medicine. During their essential general medical training, psychiatrists have correctly learned that to arrive at a diagnosis is the key to understanding whatever processes underlie the complaints and symptoms of the patient. Therefore a correct diagnosis will indicate optimal treatment and management. Unfortunately, for most patients encountered in general adult psychiatry, contemporary psychiatric knowledge does not yet extend to the identification of the processes underlying the symptoms. A syndrome takes the place of an underlying diagnosis; in other words, a list of complaints and symptoms that nowadays is called a disorder, identified by means of 'diagnostic criteria'. Logically, a case could be made for saying that both the ICD and the DSM systems are not classifications of diagnoses, but should be called 'ways of identifying disorders by means of descriptive symptoms'. Presumably the choice of the term 'diagnostic criteria' is determined largely by medical interdisciplinary pride. Psychiatrists hope to be regarded by their medical and surgical colleagues as able to do more than merely describe symptoms.

No matter how much progress is made in psychiatric classification, a cautionary note will always remain valid. Definitions and descriptions are developed on the basis of knowledge available at the time of their production and usually aim to fit the ideas and the convenience of professional workers of a particular time. This should be kept in mind because otherwise the categories of the classification may be reified. They may then become an obstacle to research and treatment, and may hinder attempts improve the classification.

Disease, illness, and sickness; a useful trio of concepts

'Disease', 'illness', and 'sickness' are often used as equivalents in ordinary conversation, but there are advantages in giving each a specific meaning in medical discourse. In this book, 'disease' will be used to indicate that there is a known abnormal physical or physiological cause for the symptoms of the patient, 'illness' for the experience of the patient, whether or not there is any understandable physical cause for the symptoms, and 'sickness' for the social consequences of the illness. There is further discussion of this important topic in Section 13.1.

Substantial changes in a classification will need to be reflected in such things as medical education, mental health legislation, and disability legislation. This may be inconvenient and troublesome, but must never be allowed to interfere with the welfare of patients and the education of mental heath professionals.

Distinguished teachers of psychiatry in the past have repeatedly taught that classification is fundamental and important (for instance within English psychiatry, Maudsley, Mapother, and Lewis in their turn all did so) but on the whole they were ignored by busy clinicians. One of the main reasons for this was probably because none of the classifications then available were of practical use. Another contributing influence was that expert classifiers did not realize how obscure their terminology seemed to the non-specialist learner. For example, the following was given as a definition of a classification by a person known to have a wide knowledge of classification in general and a serious interest in psychiatric classification in particular: 'a classification is an exhaustive set of mutually exclusive categories to aggregate data at a pre-described level of specialization for a specific purpose'. This statement is correct, and actually well put from a technical point of view, but it is not attractive or easy to understand when presented to trainee psychiatrists during a fairly intensive training session, or when translated into another language.

A problem of medical education

The topic of classification in general is not regarded as a high priority topic by those educators who construct the undergraduate curricula of modern medical schools. As expected, postgraduate courses in psychiatry usually include discussions of the categories of well-known psychiatric classifications such as Chapter V of ICD-10 and DSM-IV, but such courses rarely include considerations of how these classifications were arrived at, and their relative strengths and weaknesses.

The lack of interest in psychiatric classification was confirmed recently by a survey carried out jointly by the World Health Organization and the World Psychiatric Association in 2010 and 2011 (known as the WPA-WHO Global Survey of Psychiatrists' Attitudes towards Mental Disorders Classification); 4,887 psychiatrists in 44 countries were sent a questionnaire about their experiences with ICD-10 and hopes for ICD-11. There was a better response rate from psychiatrists in low-income countries than from high-income countries, but the overall response rate was only 34% (Reed, Mendonça Correia, et al. 2011). In other words, two-thirds of the psychiatrists were not sufficiently interested to reply.

This low status of classification as a topic in its own right must be regarded as a deficit in undergraduate and postgraduate general medical education, since the use and knowledge of internationally recognized classifications in any medical discipline is necessary for satisfactory communication between professionals. Classifications are also one of the best ways to organize contemporary knowledge about any subject that is studied in detail. For psychiatry in particular, there is also a need for a basic psychiatric classification that can be expressed in different degrees of complexity and sophistication. This was pointed out as long ago as 1938 by Aubrey Lewis,[1] but only Chapter V(F) of the ICD-10 published in 1993 has so far followed this idea.

Some of the issues considered in this book are also dealt with in Kendell's *The Role of Diagnosis in Psychiatry* (Kendell 1975). The intervening 35 years have not changed the relevance of many of the topics he covered and for the reader who wants more detail than is provided here, his book is still a valuable further resource.

A contemporary issue

Psychiatric trainees often ask 'Why is it necessary to have both ICD-10 Chapter V(F) and DSM-IV existing side by side, when the differences between them are not large?' There are several parts to the answer. The most important reason is that the World Health Organization's constitution makes the development of an international classification of diseases a mandatory function of the organization, so that all its member states are provided with a means of publishing national statistics on the morbidity and mortality rates of all types of disease. The *International Statistical Classification of Diseases and Related Health Problems* published by the World Health Organization is the means of achieving this (with periodic revisions); Chapter V has always been devoted to the psychiatric classification, now with the title of 'Mental and Behavioural Disorders.' This classification must be acceptable to the governments of all the member nations and it is only published after widespread international consultations. The governments of almost all member states (including the USA) have agreed to use it. Nevertheless, whatever national governments agree to do, professional organizations within any country are free to develop and use their own systems if they prefer and this has happened in the United Sates of America. The government of the United States of America uses the ICD, including Chapter V, for the publication of its official health statistics, but the American Psychiatric Association has always preferred to produce—for the use of its members—its own *Diagnostic and Statistical Manual of Mental Disorders* (now in its 4th edition—DSM-IV-TM). It is quite appropriate for national classifications to exist alongside the ICD, but it is helpful to all (and educational) if the reasons for this are explained and the differences between any national classifications and the ICD are listed. There is further discussion of this issue in Chapter 17.

In all the chapters, points of detail are dealt with in two ways. First, for brief comments there are footnotes to individual pages, marked by[a,b] etc. Second, for more substantial issues, indicated by a superscript number, there are longer 'chapter notes' placed at the end of each chapter. Some of the chapters and some of the more anecdotal and personal chapter notes (initialled by one of the authors) are short digressions rather than simply being additional technical information. There is a very respectable historical precedent for digressions in psychological works; Robert Burton defended his frequent use of these in *The Anatomy of Melancholy* by asserting, 'Such digressions do mightily delight and refresh a weary reader, they are like sauce to a bad stomach, and I do therefore most willingly use them.'

Some things that are not in this book

Two well-known American studies, the Stirling County study (Murphy 1994) and the Midtown Manhattan study (Srole et al. 1962) are not considered to be within the scope of this book. Both studies were unique for their time, and required a great deal of organization and hard work. But neither study made diagnosis a priority, and there was no special reference to problems of diagnostic classification.[2] In the introductory section of one of the main publications describing the NIMH Epidemiologic Catchment Area Program of the 1980s (Robins and Regier 1981) there is a brief but useful summary of these and several other large epidemiological psychiatric studies carried out in the USA between 1950 and 1980.

It has become fashionable in recent years to ask of any prominent activity, 'What is the scientific evidence for the usefulness of this?' Although in theory it is possible to design and carry out an investigation about the usefulness or cost-effectiveness of developing a psychiatric classification, a moment's reflection suggests that to spend time and resources on such a study would not be sensible. It is rather like asking a person who is about to visit a foreign country and is taking lessons in its language, 'Is there any scientific evidence that demonstrates that you should spend time and money on learning some of the language of the country before you go there?'

Notes

1 When discussing the classification of depressive states, Aubrey Lewis commented that 'The usefulness of a classification will vary according to who uses it. One that serves the clinician well may be of little value to the research worker; it may even make his task harder. The clinician wants classes into which he can put his patient's illness after a reasonably brief period of investigation, and which will assist him to make a prognosis and decide upon treatment.' (Lewis 1938). Aubrey Lewis also recommended that there should be a public health version of the classification for universal use.

2 The Stirling County study was started in 1952 by Alexander Leighton, and has continued as a very long-term follow-up study by various colleagues, particularly Jane Murphy (his wife), with some publications continuing into the 1990s. Its original primary concern was the relationship between mental disorders and social conditions in the communities under study. Three volumes have been published, Vol 1; My Name is Legion, Vol 2; People of Cove and Woodlot, and Vol 3; The Character of Danger.

The Midtown Manhattan Study (Srole et al. 1962) was not primarily concerned with psychiatric diagnoses, but with the degree of 'symptom formation', estimated by means of a questionnaire. The methods of data collection and analysis were unique to this study.

Chapter 1

Problems before agreed psychiatric classifications were available

1.1 The development of idiosyncratic ideas

In the absence of scientifically based epidemiological studies on the occurrence of severe mental illness in different countries, ideas which now seem quite bizarre and racist could gain prominence and even be discussed in reputable psychiatric journals. A good example is the idea that schizophrenia was common only in persons living in highly developed cultures (i.e. a 'disease' of modern civilization). This was closely associated with the notion that 'the African brain' was less developed than that of Europeans. As recently as 1951, a paper by Carothers was published in the *Journal of Mental Science* (the forerunner of the *British Journal of Psychiatry*) with the title 'Frontal Lobe Function in the African' (Carothers 1951). These ideas were in part a hangover effect from the rapidly diminishing British Empire, with its false assumptions about the innate superiority of the white European races. But in the absence of reliable comparative epidemiological information, these ideas—which are now seen as ridiculous—were then still regarded by some senior psychiatrists as a suitable topic for serious discussion.

1.2 Difficulties encountered by mental health professionals when trying to understand publications

1.2.1 Publications on concepts of psychiatric illness

Without an agreed way of describing the meaning of diagnostic terms, the only way to make it clear exactly what was being discussed was to include, in publications, the detailed case histories of the patients being studied. This can be satisfying for the authors, but raises problems of publishing space for editors. For instance, in a major contribution to the debate that was current in the UK in the 1930s about possible symptomatic differences between 'endogenous' and 'reactive' depressive states, Aubrey Lewis published a study based upon 61 patients that he had personally studied (Lewis 1934). This publication occupied 101 pages of the *Journal of Mental Science* but almost half of these pages were taken up by the detailed case histories of the patients. Without these details, readers would not have been able to form a useful idea of the symptoms, behaviour, and complaints of the patients.

The lack of a standard usage of diagnostic terms also meant that studies of the results of new treatments carried out in one country could not be interpreted with any confidence by psychiatrists in other countries. This problem was particularly severe in the 1940s and 1950s between the United States and most of the countries of Western Europe and was well known to senior psychiatrists who had visited or worked on both sides of the Atlantic. In the 1950s, the advent of antidepressant drugs and the widespread and successful use of electroconvulsive treatment for severe depression made the consistent use of diagnostic terms even more important and urgent. For instance, the results of the US/UK Diagnostic Project, described briefly in Chapter 2, imply that any study published in the USA in the 1940s, 1950s, and 1960s on the treatment of patients with a diagnosis of schizophrenia would be misleading for European psychiatrists. It is likely that a third—or even half—of the American patients would have been given other diagnoses in Europe (in the UK, probably some sort of affective disorder, and perhaps neurasthenia in other countries).

The extent to which classification can depend upon prejudice was demonstrated by Prince, who showed that an increase in frequency of depressive disorders closely followed the establishment of independent political states in former colonies. Prior to independence the diagnosis of depression was reserved for the colonial officers and other white persons. After independence, statistics show that the privilege of having this diagnosis was also extended to the black population (Sartorius 1973).

1.2.2 Difficulties in understanding publications on the epidemiology of psychiatric disorders

The absence of an internationally agreed classification means that the results of epidemiological studies of psychiatric disorders carried out in different countries can be compared only approximately. To take schizophrenia as an example, all the studies on the epidemiology of schizophrenia carried out before the 1980s share the problem of having some uncertainty about the diagnosis, due to not knowing the detailed grounds upon which the diagnoses were made, or who made them. Important general conclusions can, of course, often be arrived at even in the presence of some doubt about the details of the methods used; classic studies such as those of Faris and Dunham (1939), Murphy and Raman (1971), and Goldberg and Morrison (1963) all contributed something valuable in their turn. But to draw firm conclusions about possible reasons for variations in the course and outcome of the illness, or to make comparisons between different cultures, needs data of the highest possible quality. Julian Leff provides an interesting discussion on 16 studies of schizophrenia in a variety of cultures, with these limitations in mind (Leff 1981). A more recent review by Jablensky extended the discussion to 27 studies (Jablensky 2000), the more recent of which (particularly the World Health Organization Ten-Country DOSMED study (Jablensky, Sartorius, et al. 1992), used case-finding and diagnostic assessment methods that minimized the diagnostic uncertainties present in the earlier studies). Although Jablensky concludes that 'many essential questions about the nature and causes of schizophrenia still await answers', he notes that there is now firm evidence for two conclusions. First, that the clinical syndrome of schizophrenia can easily be identified in diverse populations, and this suggests that a common patho-physiology underlies the characteristic symptoms. What this common factor might be is still unknown, and the search must continue. Second, no single environmental risk factor has yet been discovered that has a major effect on the incidence of the schizophrenic syndrome. Several minor contributory influences are known, and as technology advances no doubt more will be discovered. The way they interact to produce the syndrome in each individual will presumably be the key, in the future, to a better understanding of this major international health problem, and confidence that inter-observer diagnostic variation has been minimized will be a major factor.

1.2.3 Difficulties in understanding publications on large-scale mental health statistics, particularly from other countries

Almost all countries have published information about mental hospital admissions and discharges for many years, usually under the diagnostic headings provided by the World Health Organization (WHO) in successive editions of the ICD. But unless it is made clear how such diagnoses were made and by whom, this information cannot be understood with any confidence, either within the country of origin or by psychiatrists and administrators in other countries. To illuminate these problems, large-scale studies are needed using methods of assessment that minimize the diagnostic variation between those who made the diagnoses. This was the main aim of the US/UK Diagnostic Project, described in Chapter 3.

1.3 **The proliferation of individual and national classifications**

After the Second World War, in many countries there was a marked development of all types of medical activities, including psychiatry. However, it became increasingly obvious during the 1950s that communication between psychiatrists and mental health professionals in different countries was being seriously hindered by the lack of a generally accepted way of describing psychiatric disorders. To study this problem, the WHO in Geneva commissioned Professor Erwin Stengel (Professor of Psychiatry at the University of Sheffield in the UK) to review the main psychiatric classifications then available, and to make suggestions about how to improve international communication (Stengel 1960).

Stengel illustrated what he called 'the chaotic state of the classifications in current use' by collecting 28 classifications; 11 were official, semi-official, or national classifications, and 17 that were produced on a more individual basis, but considered worthy of note. None of the 28 classifications had been published with clear definitions of the constituent terms, although the *American Classification of Mental Disorders* published by the American Psychiatric Association went some way towards this in the accompanying *Diagnostic and Statistical Manual* (DSM-II). However, most of the brief descriptions in this were described as 'reactions', so implying knowledge of aetiology. This is probably why DSM-II was not widely used outside the USA (nor was it used within the State of New York, which had its own classification).

Although almost all the member states of the United Nations had agreed to use the *International Classification of Diseases, Injuries and Causes of Death* (7th Revision) (ICD-7), only Finland, New Zealand, Peru, Thailand, and the United Kingdom actually did so. One of the reasons for this lack of enthusiasm was probably the fact that ICD-7 was simply a list of names and code numbers, with no indication of the preferred meaning of the names used. Not surprisingly, Stengel's recommendation was that an international classification should be produced by the WHO as soon as possible, accompanied by a glossary with operational definitions of its constituent categories.[1] He used the term 'operational definition' to mean information such as clear descriptions of definite symptoms and observed behaviour, without interpretations derived from any particular theory about the meaning of the symptoms. These recommendations were welcomed by the World Health Organization, and a programme of international seminars and consultations was started which led to the development of the glossary of terms to the mental health chapter of

ICD-8 (WHO 1967), and subsequent similar developments for ICD-9 and ICD-10.[3]

1.4 The facilitation of abuse of psychiatric diagnosis for political and other purposes

The abuse of psychiatric diagnoses gained prominence during the 'Cold War' when it became evident that some Soviet psychiatrists were giving psychiatric diagnoses to political dissidents, who were then admitted against their will to psychiatric institutions and given treatment (Van Voren 2010). Some of the diagnoses used depended upon syndromes that were not recognized in other countries, such as 'slowly developing schizophrenia'. This was approximately similar to 'latent schizophrenia', which made its last official appearance in ICD-8 in 1974, with the comment 'This category is not recommended for general use but a description is provided for those who believe it to be useful'. This description was 'a condition of eccentric or inconsequent behaviour and anomalies of affect that give the impression of schizophrenia though the patient has never manifested any definite and characteristic schizophrenic disturbances'. The Soviet description of this type of schizophrenia included persons who were 'stubbornly' holding on to their ideas of open dissatisfaction with the government.

The absence of internationally accepted descriptions of mental disorders also made possible the abuse of diagnoses for several other purposes, as described in *Mental Illness, Discrimination, and the Law: Fighting for Social Justice* (Callard, Sartorius, Arboleda-Flórez, et al. 2012). Sometimes a false diagnosis was used to help the patient. Thus, during the Second World War in many European countries those opposed to the regime of the occupiers were often hidden in psychiatric facilities by being given a diagnosis, while waiting for arrangements to be made to help them leave the country or join the resistance movement. Another example is that in the former Yugoslavia, patients could be helped by being given the diagnosis 'psychosis, not otherwise specified' because this meant that they were not charged for treatment while other diagnoses attracted a charge for treatment. Another more malign example was the bribing of psychiatrists by the patient's relatives eager to get at the patient's assets, to give the patient a wrong diagnosis of dementia so that they could be declared incapable of managing their own affairs.[2]

The abuse of psychiatric diagnosis for political or personal purposes needs to be distinguished from the abuse by governments of large numbers of people simply because they have a severe or long-standing mental disorder.[3] The forced labour of black people with mental disorders in South Africa is an extreme example of this type of abuse.

1.5 **Change in diagnosis caused by change in doctor**

Disagreements between clinicians about the best diagnosis for a patient's illness, even when presented with the same information, are often found in all medial specialities. Psychiatry is specially vulnerable to this problem because there are often no laboratory test results available that might make a strong case for a particular diagnosis. Anecdotal examples of this are commonplace, but an opportunity to study the problem on a large scale arose in 1964 when the results of a longitudinal study of a cohort of patients admitted for the first time to mental hospitals in England and Wales in 1954 and 1955 were published (Brooke 1963). Out of the 90,285 patients in the study, Brooke identified a subgroup of 293 who had been admitted to hospital four times during the two years of the study, and whose diagnosis as reported to the General Registrar's Office had suffered a major change at least once. Even when the admissions had all been to the same mental hospital within the two years of the study, of these 293 patients, only 37% kept the same major diagnosis throughout the two years. When the hospital case-notes of these patients were examined in detail by one psychiatrist, who applied to them a standard set of diagnostic criteria specially devised for the study—a humble forerunner of the diagnostic criteria published in 1972 by the St Louis group (Feighner et al. 1972)—the 37% rose to 81%. It was clear that a change in diagnosis was more closely associated with a change in doctor than with a change in the clinical state of the patient (Cooper 1967).

Notes

1 In 1974 The WHO published a *Glossary of Mental Disorders and Guide to their Classification* for use with ICD-8. Strictly speaking, 'glossary' means a set of explanatory notes in the margin of a document, but for want of a better term glossary has nowadays come to mean a more complete and systematic set of explanations of the meaning of terms in a document.

2 Another example was a very rich man who bribed a psychiatrist to prescribe psychotrophic drugs for his political opponent in an attempt invalidate his candidature. NS.

3 Examples of this are some of the horrors of the Second World War when thousands of the mentally ill were starved to death in occupied France or executed in Germany (von Cranach and Schneider 2010; Schneider 2011). A current form of abuse of the mentally ill by governments in a number of countries takes the form of providing a budget for the hospitalized mentally ill so low that patients die of hunger, or of coexisting physical illness for which appropriate treatment is not provided. NS.

Chapter 2

First steps towards international agreement on diagnosis and classification

2.1 The British Glossary and ICD-8

During the 1950s, a group of British senior psychiatrists became increasingly dissatisfied with the psychiatric chapter of the *7th Revision of the International Classification of Diseases*. This was little more than a list of approved names attached to a list of code numbers. At the request of the Registrar General of the UK, a committee was formed, charged with the task of producing a glossary of terms for use in the UK with the *8th Revision of the International Classification of Diseases* (due to come into operation in 1968). This was chaired by Sir Aubrey Lewis, and contained psychiatrists such as E. W. Anderson (Manchester) and E. Stengel (Sheffield), both of whom had a long-standing interest in descriptive continental psychiatry and the phenomenological approach of Jaspers.[1] The British Glossary to ICD-8 was published in 1967, and it is of interest to note that in its Introduction, there was the statement 'It is hoped that this glossary will be the first of numerous national glossaries, and the forerunner of an international glossary, which is needed in psychiatry more than in other fields of morbidity'.

A near-final draft of the British Glossary was made available to the WHO to guide the production of a glossary to Chapter V of ICD-8. Sir Aubrey Lewis and a variety of senior psychiatrists were then involved in extensive consultations with the staff of WHO Geneva over the next few years, and the final form was approved and published by WHO Geneva in 1974 with the title of *Glossary of Mental Disorders and Guide to their Classification* (WHO 1974). The foreword to this is reproduced in Appendix 1 (p. 89).

2.2 Reliable foundations for diagnosis; the Present State Examination (PSE) and the Mental Status Schedule (MSS)

To be reliable and useful, a diagnosis needs to rest on a secure basis of symptoms that have been clearly described in adequate detail. ('Symptom' is used here to mean psychological and behavioural phenomena which are generally thought by psychiatrists to be indicative of mental illnesses.) During the 1950s, a number of symptom rating scales was published in the international literature, all with the same basic aim of making it convenient for researchers to have a systematic record of symptoms in the patients under study. However, they differed widely in the number and details of the symptoms covered, and none was accompanied either by recommendations about the style of interviewing, or by detailed descriptions of what was meant by their constituent symptoms. Two such rating scales, still used occasionally, are Hamilton's Rating Scale for Depression, which occupies only one page, covering 16 symptoms (Hamilton 1960) and Overall and Gorham's Brief Psychiatric Rating Scale, which occupies several pages, covering many symptoms each rated on a seven-point scale. (Overall and Gorham 1962). Neither of these early rating scales are accompanied by instructions, and it is left to the user to decide how to define the symptoms, and whether to interview the patient or not.

To use any published symptom rating schedule was certainly better than simply stating the diagnosis of the patients studied, but the first generation of rating scales still left a great deal unsaid. So, during the early 1960s, John Wing and his colleagues in the Social Psychiatry Unit at the Institute of Psychiatry in London decided to reduce inter-psychiatrist variation as much as possible by producing a symptom rating system in which the interviewing style was also specified, and in which all the symptoms were described in detail in an accompanying glossary. From the start, the intention was to produce a research procedure, so it was likely to be too detailed and lengthy for daily routine use in busy clinical settings. It was also assumed that the resulting procedure would be used in research projects carried out by a team of investigators, who would first attend a course of instruction in its use, and then practice together until a satisfactory standard of inter-rater agreement was achieved.

All the symptoms currently regarded as indicative of mental illness, and a number of other non-diagnostic symptoms important to the patients, such as muscular tension and worrying, were brought together in an interviewing and rating schedule to form the Present State Examination (PSE) (Wing, Birley, Cooper, et al. 1967; Wing, Cooper, and Sartorius 1974). An interviewing style closely resembling ordinary clinical questioning was also specified.[2] Each symptom is defined in an accompanying glossary, which the interviewer is required to learn before starting to interview patients for study.

The PSE system is probably the most comprehensive of all the symptom rating schedules available and, following its adoption by the WHO, now exists in many languages and has been used in many countries and cultures.

Early versions of the PSE were used in the US/UK Diagnostic Project and the International Pilot Study of Schizophrenia (IPSS) of the WHO, and the 10th Revision forms the central part of the Schedules for the Clinical Assessment of Neuropsychiatry (SCAN) (Wing, Babor, Brugha, et al. 1990).

Because of its comprehensive content, a SCAN interview with a subject who has some sort of psychiatric disorder usually takes around 30–45 minutes or even longer. This contrasts with the 15 minutes or so needed to complete SCAN with a normal subject with no symptoms. An experienced psychiatrist not using any form of structured interview, whose purpose is only to establish the main diagnosis, is likely to find the main symptoms quickly and be able to finish the interview more quickly than a SCAN interviewer.

There are two common misunderstandings about the PSE (and its successor SCAN). First, that the interview and rating procedure produces a diagnosis, and second, that its use is necessarily accompanied by the 'category fallacy' of Kleinman (that is, an imposition of culturally determined assumptions about the diagnosis (Kleinman 1987)). Anybody who studies the details of the origin of the PSE or attends a PSE/SCAN training course quickly realizes that these are elementary misunderstandings. The interviewing and rating procedures produce a list of symptoms that are based upon the experience of the patient, interviewed in the appropriate native language. It is entirely up to the researcher to decide how to use these symptoms, and whether they will be used to contribute to a diagnosis. A set of computer programs is now available, if required, which use the symptoms to produce both ICD-10 and DSM-IV diagnoses, but use of these is entirely optional.

At about the same time as the PSE was being developed in London, the Mental Status Schedule (MSS) was independently produced by R. Spitzer and colleagues at the Biometrics Department of the New York State Psychiatric Institute (Spitzer, Fleiss, et al. 1964). This had the same general aim as the PSE, in that it produced a description of the symptoms of the patient, but it had significant differences. The MSS contained fewer symptoms than the PSE, and many were rated in not so much detail. In addition, the interviewer was required to follow the exact wording and order of the questions as printed in the schedule. The MSS was quickly followed by the Psychiatric State Schedule (PSS), whose content was much closer to that of the PSE, but still required the interviewer to follow exactly the wording and order of the questions in the schedule. (Spitzer, Endicott, et al. 1970). Spitzer and colleagues also wrote a computer program DIAGNO, which produces the most likely DSM-II diagnosis when the MSS symptoms are entered (Spitzer and Endicott 1968). This was the first computer program available that removes an important source of human variation in the diagnostic process, but inevitably has built into it the diagnostic preferences of whoever writes the program (and the same applies to the CATEGO programs that give the output from the PSE/SCAN system). DIAGNO was used in the US/UK project to check the consistency of the study project diagnoses made in New York and London before the program CATEGO for the PSE was written.

Because of its more flexible interviewing style and its more comprehensive coverage of symptoms, the PSE system was adopted by the WHO for use in its International Pilot Study of Schizophrenia (IPSS).

Notes

1 Professors Anderson and Stengel were both noted for their wide clinical knowledge, but their expertise was equalled by their tenacity of opinions and irascible temperaments. Professor Ken Rawnsley was the secretary to this committee, and had many fascinating anecdotes to tell of the lively meetings. JEC.

2 The PSE is a semi-structured interviewing procedure which covers a comprehensive set of symptoms, allied to a detailed glossary which defines each symptom. A set of computer programs is also available which condenses the symptoms rated, first into syndromes and then into categories, as an aid to diagnosis. Each section of the interview starts with an obligatory question about a symptom, which is then followed up by further questions at the interviewer's discretion, depending upon the patient's reply. The PSE is designed for use by professional mental health workers in research studies, after an intensive one-week training course.

Chapter 3
Large-scale collaborative studies on diagnosis

3.1 Cross-national: The US/UK Diagnostic Project

The disparities between American and European diagnostic concepts noted in Section 1.2 were well known to the senior psychiatrists of most countries, but the only studies that had been carried out by the early 1960s on this problem were on a comparatively small scale (Sandifer et al. 1968, Katz et al. 1969). There was still no body of reliable clinical evidence of sufficient size upon which to base constructive discussions and possible solutions.

So a group in the USA, led by Morton Kramer (Chief of Biometry, National Institute of Mental Health, Washington, USA) and Joseph Zubin (Head of Biometrics Research, New York State Dept of Mental Hygiene, Columbia University, New York), initiated a large-scale project to be funded by the National Institute of Mental Health (NIMH) of the USA to study the reasons for these problems on a larger scale. The first stage used available national hospital admission statistics to illustrate the problems, and the second stage involved a more detailed study of the diagnoses given to large numbers of individual patients, conducted in several hospitals in New York and London.

3.1.1 Large-scale national statistics of admissions to mental hospitals

Kramer (1961, 1969) showed that although the total first admission rates for adults with all types of mental illness in the USA and in England and Wales were reasonably similar: (1) the first admission rate for schizophrenia in England and Wales was about one third lower than in the United States; (2) the first admission rate for manic-depressive illness in England and Wales was nine times higher than that in the U.SA; and (3) the first admission rate for psychosis with arteriosclerosis in England and Wales was about one-tenth that in the USA.

3.1.2 **Detailed study of individual diagnoses**

After discussions with Professors Aubrey Lewis and Michael Shepherd of the Institute of Psychiatry in London, a large grant was obtained from the National Institute of Mental Health (NIMH) in Washington in 1963 to study the problem in detail, with Joseph Zubin as the principal investigator.[1] The resulting US/UK Diagnostic Project, whose teams of investigators were able to interchange between London and New York, demonstrated that almost all of the diagnostic differences of the type noted above were due to differences between the diagnostic opinions of hospital psychiatrists, rather than the result of differences between the clinical states of the patients upon whom the official hospital diagnoses were based (Cooper, Kendell, Gurland, Sartorius, et al. 1969; Cooper, Kendell, Gurland, et al. 1972). A summary of some of the results of the US/UK Diagnostic Project is given in Appendix 2.

The staff of the diagnostic project also did another type of study in which videotapes of selected patients were shown to audiences of British and American psychiatrists who made whatever diagnoses they thought appropriate. These videotape studies can be thought of as keeping the stimulus (i.e. the patient) constant while allowing the response (i.e. the psychiatric assessments) to vary. In the videotape studies, the same type of diagnostic differences between British and American psychiatrists were found that were present in the hospital admission studies (Kendell, Copeland, et al. 1971).

Videotaped case-presentations later became a routine part of the WHO Programme on Standardization of Psychiatric Diagnosis.

3.2 **International: The WHO Programmes on the Standardization of Psychiatric Diagnosis and Classification; Programmes A, B, C, and D**

In the years after the Second World War, public health issues received considerable attention across the world, and some important aspects of psychiatry were often included. In part this was due to the war-time success which some mass health measures (such as screening and disinfection) had enjoyed, and in part to the optimism and belief in the possibilities of a better future that seem to follow major wars. This was an optimism that made it possible to believe that some diseases, such as malaria, syphilis, and tuberculosis, could be eradicated, and many others controlled. The result was a number of good years for public health programmes in many countries extending into the early 1960s; these years were marked by an enthusiastic acceptance of health planning, discussion of the possibility of epidemiological surveillance of diseases, and the initiation of disease eradication programmes.

The World Health Organization was at the forefront of many of these efforts, and its leadership saw public health issues, such as methods for epidemiological investigations and techniques for health service planning, as its contribution to the development of national health programmes (Sartorius 2002). The first publication showing the interest of the WHO in the field of mental health was the report by Professor Erwin Stengel on the chaotic state of psychiatric classifications (already discussed in Section 1.3). WHO also sponsored the publication of a booklet by Professor D.D. Reid, *Epidemiological Methods in the Study of Mental Disorders,* which is still a good starting place for anyone wanting a clearly written introduction to the techniques and methods of psychiatric epidemiology (Reid 1960). Reid was not a psychiatrist, but had a rare combination of expertise in general medical epidemiology and a sympathetic approach to the special problems of psychiatry. This was followed by a complementary WHO publication, *The Scope of Epidemiology in Psychiatry* (Lin and Standley 1962).

The WHO also engaged experts as visiting WHO consultants who advised a number of countries on ways of improving statistical reporting and designing mental health care programmes. WHO has always had in mind the important differences between clinical psychiatry, and the development of mental health programmes of a much broader nature. Mental health programmes are aggregates of activities designed to (i) promote mental health; (ii) prevent mental illness; (iii) ensure the treatment of the mentally ill; (iv) rehabilitate those who are disabled by mental disorders; and (v) provide technical support to efforts that aim to diminish psychosocial problems, such as violence and the erosion of family life in conditions of rapid social change (WHO 1992a; Sartorius 2002).[3]

During the early 1960s, Tsung-yi Lin was responsible for epidemiological and social psychiatry in the WHO Mental Health Unit, and after extensive consultations with leaders of psychiatry in many countries, a programme was produced (with the publication of ICD-9 in mind, due in 1975) that had four components planned as an overlapping sequence of complementary activities. It was intended from the start that the staff of WHO would as usual initiate and coordinate the various activities, but also be directly involved in some of the work. This direct involvement of WHO staff was unusual, but it remained a valuable feature of the Mental Health Division for many years.

These four programmes, labelled A, B, C, and D, were based upon the development of

1. a classification of mental disorders that would be internationally acceptable
2. standardized procedures for case-finding and for the assessment of the severity of the illness

3. a core of trained research personnel

4. a network of research centres for the exchange of research data, ideas and skills, and also for training (Lin 1967).

Programme A was a series of eight international seminars at yearly intervals, all of which were attended by a core group of 12 experts from different schools of psychiatry, plus a variety of additional experts from each host centre in turn. The first seminar in London in 1965 on 'Functional Psychoses' was organized by Professor Michael Shepherd, and used both written case histories and videotape recordings (Shepherd, Brooke, et al. 1968) This was probably the first use of videotaped interviews in the UK.[2] The other seminars covered the following topics: 1966 (Oslo) Borderline psychoses and reactive psychoses; 1967 (Paris) Psychiatric disorders of childhood; 1968 (Moscow) Mental disorders of old age; 1969 (Washington) Mental retardation; 1970 (Basle) Neurotic disorders and psychosomatic disorders; 1971 (Tokyo) Personality disorders and drug addiction; 1972 (Geneva) Summary, conclusions, recommendations, and proposals for further research.

Programme B was the setting up of cross-cultural methods of assessment and diagnosis so as to test the practical application of some of the diagnostic concepts being developed in Programme A. This would also test whether the criteria agreed upon for particular disorders could be uniformly applied in different countries of contrasting cultures and differing schools of psychiatry by means of standardized symptom rating procedures. The first such study was the International Pilot Study of Schizophrenia (IPSS) carried out in eight Field Research Centres (FRCs) (in Colombia, Czechoslovakia, Denmark, India, Nigeria, Union of Soviet Socialist Republics, United Kingdom, and United States of America). This study is described later in Chapter 5, Section 5.1. An important aspect of the IPSS was the establishment of the network of FRCs, in the hope that these would serve as training centres for the much needed research and teaching staff for other collaborative studies in the future, that would constitute the elements of Programme C.

Programme C This was to be a comprehensive epidemiological study of defined mental disorders in geographically defined populations. It was anticipated that Programme B would need some time to be established, so a gap of several years between the two was considered likely. In the event, Programme C took the form of the study called the Determinants of Outcome of Severe Mental Disorders (DOSMED), designed in 1975–6 and started in an expanded network of FRCs in 1978. This is described later in Chapter 5, Section 5.2.

Programme D Training programmes in epidemiological research techniques. These took several forms over a period of approximately ten years.

First, small groups of WHO postgraduate fellows spent defined periods of time at some of the FRCs (such as Aarhus, Groningen, London, and Mannheim). In addition, two international workshops were organized by WHO Geneva (Tehran in 1975 and Khartoum in 1977) that resulted in a publication intended as an aid to the planning of future seminars and postgraduate courses (Baasher et al. 1982).The final phase of Programme D was a series of seminars organized jointly between the Division of Mental Health, WHO Geneva, and the Ministry of Health of the People's Republic of China, in 1980, 1981, and 1982. These were a boost to postgraduate psychiatric education in China, which was starting up again after the difficult period of isolation and internal strife of the 'cultural revolution' which ended around 1979 (Cooper 1982a).

The overall programme also had other parts, such as the production of a glossary of mental disorders, already described, produced with the help of Sir Aubrey Lewis and a variety of other advisors, such as Professors Anderson and Stengel.[3] The glossary was included alongside the headings and codes of the mental health Chapter V of ICD-8 in the main ICD volumes; this was unusual for its time but was accepted as reasonable by the ICD unit in view of the special problems for psychiatry caused by the relative scarcity of independent measures to guide the diagnostic progress.

In addition, a tri-axial classification of disorders of childhood was drafted by M. Rutter in collaboration with L. Eisenberg and M. Shepherd, for presentation at a meeting of the Programme A group in Paris in 1976 (Rutter et al. 1969 and 1975). This proved to be popular, and served as a basis for the multi-axial classification of disorders of childhood that was prepared to accompany the ICD-10. The videotaped case presentations and the written case history assessments (used for these programmes in many countries for the first time) also were an important demonstration of convenient methods of how to study agreement and disagreement between clinicians; they were often subsequently used in the widespread exercises needed to produce Chapter V of ICD-10 (Shepherd, Brooke, et al. 1968).

Notes

1 There was also a US steering committee, composed of Dr Morton Kramer and Professors Joseph Zubin, Paul Hoch, and Benjamin Pasamanik, whose functions were unspecified but generally helpful. JEC.

2 Professor Michael Shepherd was the first in the UK to realize the practical advantages of videotape over cinefilm. The first generation of videotape machines were formidable, in that they were large, gave off a good deal of heat and noise, and employed tape that was two inches wide, that had to go round a rapidly whirling cylindrical recording head. Fortunately, by the time the

US/UK Diagnostic Project started, the more user-friendly Ampex one-inch tape machines were available in the USA, and one was imported for use in the UK side of the Diagnostic Project. A special current converter was needed to change the UK 50 cycle mains electricity to the 60 cycles required for the machine. JEC.

3 Psychiatrists are sometimes leaders of mental health programmes, but this is not necessarily always the case. The fund of knowledge upon which a mental health programme is based must always have psychiatry as a large component, but having such knowledge is not by itself a sufficient qualification for a programme leader. The multitude of activities that must be included in comprehensive mental health programmes is such that the skills and knowledge of experts ranging from anthropologists and economists to practitioners of biological sciences and philosophy need to be involved in the planning and implementation of these programmes. Successful builders of mental health programmes have usually been successful because of their leadership qualities and not because of their mastery of psychiatry and allied sciences. NS.

Chapter 4

Developments in the USA

4.1 The DSM system

4.1.1 DSM-I and DSM-II

The need to assess the mental state of large numbers of military personnel in World War II led to the production of psychiatric classification schemes by the Office of the Surgeon General, called at first 'Medical 203'. Following the publication in 1949 by the World Health Organization of the sixth revision of the International Statistical Classification of Diseases (ICD), which for the first time included a section on mental disorders, the American Psychiatric Association produced an updated and extended version of Medical 203, under the title of *The Diagnostic and Statistical Manual*, published in 1952 (DSM-I). The eighth revision of the ICD, published by the WHO in 1968, stimulated the APA to produce another version, DSM-II, under the chairmanship of Ernest Gruenberg. Both DSM-I and DSM-II reflected the psychodynamic approach to psychiatry that was then predominant in the USA, and symptoms typifying mental disorders were not described in detail.

There were, however, some exceptions to this overall psychodynamic trend, particularly at Washington University in St Louis, Kansas (Professor Eli Robins), and in New York at the Biometrics Department of the New York State Psychiatric Institute (Professor Joseph Zubin).

4.2 The St Louis group and the Feighner criteria

The St Louis group (notably Eli Robins, George Winokur, and Sam Guze) developed an interest in descriptive diagnosis, genetics, and the possible biological basis of mental disorders that in the USA is sometimes called the neo-Kraepelinian movement. An important publication from this group gave in detail a set of 'diagnostic criteria for research' (Feighner, Robins, Guze, et al. 1972), and they also collaborated with the Biometrics Department to produce similar publications (Spitzer, Endicott, and Robins 1975).

4.3 **DSM-III**

The chairman of the DSM-II Task Force, Ernest Gruenberg, had taken care to ensure that its basic structure and headings followed that of ICD-7, so DSM-II had been an improvement on DSM-I. In spite of this important change, DSM-II had only limited appeal and use, even within the USA. This was probably due to the brevity of the purely narrative paragraphs of description of each category.

When the time came for the preparation of DSM-III, it was not surprising that Spitzer was appointed as overall chairman of the process. Many working parties, task forces, and committees were needed for the task. Lists of descriptive diagnostic criteria were prepared for each disorder, and there were extensive field trials of these, involving several hundred psychiatrists in the USA. The resulting DSM-III was published as a full-sized book, containing a narrative description of the clinical features of each disorder, plus a list of detailed diagnostic criteria (APA 1980a). DSM-III was also published as a pocket book and as a mid-sized Desk Reference version; these latter two containing only the lists of diagnostic criteria. (APA 1980b).Within a year, the pocket–sized quick reference book had sold more than 100,000 copies.[1]

The novel approach of the content and terminology of DSM-III is illustrated by the complete omission of such familiar terms as neurosis and hysteria. These words are not even in the index to the main volume. This radically different DSM-III, clearly giving precedence to the needs of researchers, was not welcomed by many members of the American Psychiatric Association, a large proportion of whom were clinicians not engaged in research. Despite some opposition, it was finally approved by the APA Board of Trustees, and so began a new era of potentially improved precision in psychiatric diagnosis.

DSM-III was certainly welcomed by editors of major psychiatric journals, because its use produces a step-change in the extent to which research publications can be understood. The use of lists of diagnostic criteria has great advantages for research, where usually the researcher has adequate information and time specially allotted to making diagnoses, but the situation can be very different for busy clinicians. Further discussion of the pros and cons of reliance upon lists of diagnostic criteria can be found in Sections 14.4 and 14.5.

4.4 **DSM-III-R, DSM-IV, and DSM-IV-TR**

DSM-III-R followed in 1987, DSM-IV in 1994, and DSM-IV-TR in 2000. DSM-III-R and DSM-IV contained many changes of detail but no radical differences in the general style and approach of the original DSM-III.

(See comments on the publication of DSM-IV; Cooper 1995.) At the time of writing, DSM-IV-TR is the current version, published in 2000. TR (text revision) indicates that a small number of revisions of the textual description of the disorders were thought to be justified, without changing the details of the criteria.

Note

1 Table 4.1 shows the number of copies printed of the Quick Reference to the Diagnostic Criteria from DSM-III.

Table 4.1 Number of copies printed of the Quick Reference to the Diagnostic Criteria from DSM-III

First printing	25,000 copies	Feb 1980
Second printing	30,000 copies	May 1980
Third printing	40,000 copies	September 1980
Fourth printing	30,000 copies	December 1980
Fifth printing	40,000 copies	March 1981
Sixth printing	20,000 copies	August 1982
Seventh printing	35,000 copies	May 1983
Eighth printing	25,000 copies	June 1984

Chapter 5

The first internationally understandable epidemiological studies

5.1 The IPSS and DOSMED studies of the WHO

The development of the improved symptom rating and diagnostic methods that made the US/UK Diagnostic Project possible also meant that other and more extensive cross-cultural comparisons of psychiatric disorders could be carried out. The International Pilot Study of Schizophrenia (IPSS), initiated by Tsung-yi Lin of WHO Geneva, was the first of a number of such studies (Lin 1967; WHO 1975).

This started in 1967, and was very successful, partly because its original aims were quite modest, and clearly formulated. These were set out as;

1. The devising of standard research instruments and procedures for case-finding, and for the degree of psychiatric impairment in schizophrenia.

2. The demonstration that comparable cases of schizophrenic disorders can be identified in different cultures.

3. the demonstration that psychiatrists in different countries can use standardized assessment instruments and make reliable diagnoses.

4. The description of the course taken by cases in the period after their firm diagnosis.

In 1965, Tsung-yi Lin obtained the cooperation of teams of investigators in eight Field Research Centres (FRC) in Aarhus (Denmark), Cali (Columbia), Agra (India), Ibadan (Nigeria), Taipei (Taiwan), Washington (USA), and London (UK).[1] A 9th, Prague (Czechoslovakia), was added in 1967.

Most of the FRCs in countries where English was not the first language had at least two investigators who spoke English and most of them had an investigator who had had at least some of their postgraduate psychiatric education in the UK or the USA. The FRCs represented developed and developing countries, as well as countries from both the East and West of

Europe, and it was considered that the final group contained an adequate diversity of cultures and service systems for a pilot study. The Present State Examination (8th edition) was chosen for assessment of the mental state, and other schedules were devised to cover the history, social, and family aspects of the patients. All the FRCs coped well with the necessary translations and modifications of the interviewing and rating schedules, enabling the study to proceed on timetable, as planned.

In each FRC a 'convenience sample' of 120 patients was brought into the study. These were patients aged 15–45 years who contacted defined psychiatric facilities, who satisfied inclusion criteria suggestive of a psychiatric illness, such as hallucinations, delusions, and inexplicable behaviour, and who did not have exclusion criteria (such as symptoms suggestive of traumatic brain damage). The final study group totaled 1,202 patients, divided more or less equally between the nine centres. Their clinical state was recorded using a slightly modified version of the 8th edition of the Present State Examination and other specially prepared schedules. It soon became clear that patients suffering from both acute and long-lasting 'typical' schizophrenic syndromes could easily be found in all the FRCs. A major innovative feature of the IPSS was that each year, a meeting of two investigators from all the FRCs, with a few external study advisors, was held in each FRC in turn. This was useful for the FRC because it drew attention to the fact that the FRC was participating in a major WHO study, and emphasized to the local authorities the importance of developing mental health services. It also helped to create and maintain a unique network of centres with shared professional skills and continuing personal relationships between the investigators. This was of great value for the IPSS and for the development of other subsequent WHO collaborative studies.

The two-year and five-year follow-up of the patients in each of the FRCs produced an unexpected finding; in the FRCs in the so-called 'developing' countries (Agra in India, Ibadan in Nigeria, and Cali in Colombia), higher proportions of patients with a diagnosis of schizophrenia fell into the good outcome categories than in other 'developed' centres such as London, Moscow, and Aarhus.

5.2 The WHO Determinants of Outcome of Severe Mental Disorders (DOSMED) study

The puzzling finding just noted was one of the principal motivations for the World Health Organization to set up the subsequent epidemiologically-based study of the Determinants of Outcome of Severe Mental Disorders (DOSMED) (Jablensky, Sartorius, et al. 1992).[2]

For this study, a wider set of cultures was covered by the addition of FRCs in Chandigarh (India), Nagasaki (Japan), Honolulu (USA), and Dublin (Ireland). In the UK, Nottingham replaced London. Each FRC defined a catchment area of at least several hundred thousand persons aged 15–54 years, from which all persons who developed a new (lifetime first) potentially schizophrenic illness were assessed and included in a two-year follow-up study. Special arrangements were made to prevent 'leakage' of new cases of schizophrenia, so as to obtain data as close as possible to the 'administrative incidence' of schizophrenia for the follow-up study. The two main findings of the DOSMED study were: (1) a confirmation of the better outcome for people with typical schizophrenic illness in the developing centres; and (2) that the incidence of schizophrenia is surprisingly similar (although by no means identical) in all the FRCs when compared with the very wide variations in incidence found for many physical disorders.

5.3 The International Study of Schizophrenia (ISOS)

These findings were confirmed again by the latest WHO report published as the International Study of Schizophrenia (ISOS) (Hopper, Harrison, Janca, and Sartorius 2007). In this, the IPSS and the DOSMED data are put together with data from a number of other similar studies sponsored by the WHO, to give follow-up assessment on a total of more than 1,000 patients in 14 countries, over follow-up periods of 15–20 years. The reason for this better outcome in the FRCs in the developing (i.e. comparatively non-industrialized) countries is still not understood. Speculations are possible (Cooper and Sartorius 1977), but as yet no explanation based on data or new studies has been forthcoming.

The DOSMED findings are also relevant to the current debates (stimulated by the preparations for ICD-11 and DSM-V) about the usefulness of the concept of schizophrenia, and of the traditional distinction between the schizophrenic syndromes and the manic-depressive psychoses. In the DOSMED study, relapses in patients with both these original diagnoses run true to type far more often than not, and the outcome within the study population for patients with schizophrenia was much less favourable than for the smaller number of patients with severe affective illness. In addition, in all the study areas, the age- and gender-specific curves of incidence follow a similar pattern, and there is a general tendency for the onset of schizophrenia to occur later in females than in males.

Notes

1 Taipei had to be later excluded from the study because of the recognition of Beijing as the capital of China. This meant that, according to WHO protocol, correspondence with Taipei would have to have been channelled via Beijing, which was unacceptable to the authorities in Taiwan. The Taiwan data plus follow-up studies have been published independently, and are not included in the WHO publications of the overall follow-up studies. NS.

2 Preparations for the IPSS were helped in some important respects by the staff of the US/UK Diagnostic Project (Cooper et al. 1969, 1972; Kramer 1969; Zubin 1969). These two studies were quite separate administratively and financially, although both were aimed at clarifying cross-cultural and cross-national problems associated with the diagnostic process and major mental illnesses. The team of the US/UK study (which included N. Sartorius as one of the main interviewers in the first Netherne-Brooklyn hospital admissions study) carried out some joint training interviews with the principal investigators of the IPSS centres, using the mobile caravan videotape studio already developed by the US/UK team at the Institute of Psychiatry in London. These two overlapping studies owed a great deal to the administrative support and financial influence of Dr Morton Kramer of the National Institute of Mental Health of the USA. JEC.

Chapter 6

Large community-based diagnostic studies in the USA

6.1 The NIMH Epidemiological Catchment Areas Programme (ECA) (1982–1983)

DSM-III had been published in 1980, so it was then of great interest to know how persons with its constituent disorders were distributed in the population, including persons in hospitals and other institutions. The National Institute of Mental Health therefore decided to fund a large community survey, whose major objective was 'to obtain prevalence rates of specific mental disorders as defined by DSM-III', in the hope of improving 'our understanding of etiology, clinical course, and response to treatment of any specific disorder' (Regier et al. 1984). Another aim was 'to identify treated and untreated prevalence rates of both the severe mental disorders, found in higher concentrations in institutions, and the less severe disorders, found more frequently in communities'.

The full title of this series of studies is *The National Institute of Mental Health Multisite Epidemiologic Catchment Area (ECA) Program in the USA*. It was carried out in five areas, each containing a well-known research centre; these were: Baltimore (Johns Hopkins University); St Louis, Kansas (Washington University); Durham, North Carolina (Duke University); New Haven, Connecticut (Yale University); and Los Angeles (University of California, Neuropsychiatric Institute). Most of the interviewing in these five areas was carried out in 1981 and 1982. The total sample size was about 25,000, with at least 3,500 subjects per site, thus making it the largest survey of its type ever carried out in the USA. The large sample size was necessary to ensure that reasonable numbers of persons with disorders with expected frequencies of around 1% of the population (such as schizophrenic disorders) would be included in the study.

Diagnostic assessment was by means of the Diagnostic Interview Schedule (DIS). This was a development of an earlier schedule, the Renard Diagnostic Interview, that covered the St Louis (Feighner) criteria. Further modifications were made by Lee Robins and colleagues of St Louis, to ensure coverage of DSM-III diagnoses, so producing the DIS. This was designed to be administered by specially trained lay interviewers rather than by psychiatrists (Robins, Helzer, et al. 1981; Robins, Helzer, Ratcliff, et al. 1982).

The questions in the DIS covered the presence, duration, and severity of individual symptoms. Using these questions, the interviewer first determined whether the symptom ever occurred, then its severity in terms of any limitation of activities. There were then questions as to whether a doctor or other professional has been consulted about it, whether medication has been taken as treatment, and whether it could be explained by medical illness, alcohol, or other drug intake. Symptoms that met the severity criteria and that were not completely explained by medical conditions or substances ingested were rated as present. The interviewers (preferably experienced market research interviewers) went through an intensive two-week training course, in which there was a great deal of personal supervision by experienced interviewers.

The DIS did not require the interviewer to make any decisions concerning the existence or non-existence of a psychiatric disorder. The interviewer read specific questions, and followed positive responses with additional prescribed questions. Each step in the sequence of identifying a psychiatric symptom was fully specified and did not depend upon the judgement of the interviewer. All the symptom questions are asked of all respondents. There was no skipping out of a section after a few negative answers suggested that the person would not meet diagnostic criteria.

The DIS did not cover all 122 adult diagnoses in DSM-III, but included the 20 that were regarded as the most common and most important.

6.2 **The results of the ECA programme**

This is not the place to discuss the results of the ECA for individual disorders in detail, which can be found in the many publications that subsequently appeared during the 1980s. But it is reassuring to note that for most disorders, the findings were of the same order of magnitude as might have been anticipated. For instance, a roughly 1% lifetime expectancy of one or other of the schizophrenic syndromes was found, and around 15–20% of the population were found to be experiencing some sort of anxiety or depression. An important finding was that disorders often occur together at a rate well above chance (called 'co-occurrence' or 'co-morbidity'). For instance, 18% of the total population, or 60% of those with at least one disorder, had had at least two psychiatric disorders in their lifetime. Of even greater interest than lifetime co-occurrence is co-occurrence within the last year, which indicates how often people suffer from multiple disorders simultaneously.

Co-occurrence must mean shared symptoms, shared risk factors, or that one disorder causes another. These possibilities are discussed in detail in the major publications arising from the ECA study, such as Robins and Regier (Eds) 1981 (Robins, Helzer, et al. 1984).

A major point to be remembered in all the discussions of co-occurrence is that the abuse of and dependence upon alcohol and drugs are frequently involved. These are, of course, general and mental health problems of major and international importance, but many psychiatrists regard them as being of a different nature to morbid states of anxiety, depression, and the psychoses. Although it may be administratively and politically convenient to include them as a part of psychiatry, as is usually done at the moment, in a more rational world, disorders due directly to alcohol and drugs would deserve their own specialist organizations and services.

The ECA study was a major practical achievement, in that it showed that large-scale community surveys could be conducted in the USA by using specially trained lay interviewers. The high rate of co-occurrence of disorders, plus the fact that the ECA study was confined to specific regions, stimulated the next major survey in the USA some ten years later, the National Co-Morbidity Survey (Kessler, McGonagle, et al. 1994) and ten years after that, the NIMH National Co-Morbidity Replication Survey (Kessler, Berglund, et al. 2004); these are described briefly in the next section.

6.3 The NIMH National Co-Morbidity Survey (1990–1992) and the NIMH National Co-Morbidity Replication Survey (2001–2003)

The first of these two surveys was conducted on a national probability sample of 8,098 civilian, non-institutionalized subjects aged 15–54 years, and the interview used was the successor to the DIS, the Composite International Diagnostic Interview (CIDI) (Kessler, McGonagle, et al. 1994). The WHO version of the CIDI was modified for this study for several reasons, one of which was so that the results could be expressed in terms of DSM-III-R, the revised edition of the DSM. Although the lifetime and 12-month prevalence rates of disorders were fairly close to those found in the ECA study, most rates were somewhat higher. Nearly 50% of respondents reported at least one lifetime disorder, and close to 30% reported at least one 12-month disorder. The most common disorders were major depressive episode, alcohol dependence, social phobia, and simple phobia. The authors concluded that 'the prevalence of psychiatric disorders is greater than previously thought to be the case. Furthermore, this morbidity is more highly concentrated than previously recognized in roughly one sixth of the population who have a history of three or more psychiatric disorders'. Another striking finding was that the majority of people with psychiatric disorders fail to obtain professional treatment. Even among people with a lifetime history of three or more comorbid disorders, the proportion who ever obtain specialty sector mental health treatment is less that 50%.

These findings were confirmed ten years later by means of the The National Co-Morbidity Replication Survey (2001–3) using similar methods and 9,282 participants. (Kessler, Berglund, Chiu, et al. 2004).

The results of these large surveys illustrate the difference between a person who receives a diagnosis, and a person who is a 'case' in the sense of contacting the services asking for help, but who may not have all the symptoms specified as being necessary to receive a diagnosis.

Chapter 7

Other large community-based diagnostic surveys

7.1 The Chinese National Epidemiological Survey of Mental Disorders (1982)

This nationwide epidemiological survey of mental disorders in the People's Republic of China was completed in 1982, after collaboration over several years between the psychiatric teams working in the 12 participating centres. Professor Shen Yucun (Beijing) was chair of the overall coordinating committee. The teams received technical advice and support from both the Regional Office of the World Health Organization in Manila and the Division of Mental Health of the World Health Organization in Geneva. The survey measured the point prevalence of mental disorders, including mental handicap. This survey was of unique importance for China, because it involved the use of modern standardized methods of assessment by Chinese psychiatrists, and because it was the first large-scale national survey of mental disorders using such methods in China. The 12 centres were chosen so as to have differing geographical and sociocultural environments, and each centre studied both a rural and an urban sample of 500 households each. The 12,000 households that comprised the total sample studied contained 51,982 persons (38,136 over the age of 15 years). The Chinese originators of the study were keen from the start to assess the subjects in the study by means of the 9th edition of the Present State Examination (Wing et al. 1974), in spite of the extensive training of survey psychiatrists that would be necessary. This would allow them to make conventional psychiatric diagnoses in the European descriptive style of psychiatry with which they were already familiar (because many of the senior Chinese psychiatrists had experienced postgraduate psychiatric education in the Soviet Union).

A number of papers giving the results of the survey were published in Chinese in the *Chinese Journal of Neurology and Psychiatry* in 1986 and 1987, but it was not until 1990 that 12 drafts in English became available, that could be brought together to form an adequate description of the study for publication outside China. Following visits in 1990 to Beijing, Nanjing,

Shanghai, and Harbin in 1990 to discuss the survey with the staff of some of the survey centres and to obtain further data, an account of the survey was published in English in 1996 (Cooper and Sartorius 1996). The details of the survey methods and its findings are given in the publication, but it is worth noting here that some of the rates (for instance for schizophrenia) are quite similar to those reported by studies using the same methods in other countries. Some other rates (for instance, for neurotic and depressive disorders) are markedly lower.

7.2 In the UK: The OPCS Survey of Psychiatric Morbidity in Great Britain

This was a study of the prevalence of psychiatric morbidity among adults aged 16–64, living in private households, in Great Britain. It had an unusual focussed design, in that between April 1993 and August 1944, four separate surveys were carried out on persons aged between 16–64 years:

(i)   10,000 adults living in private households.

(ii) 350 persons with psychosis living in private households.

(iii) 1,200 persons living in institutions specifically catering for people with mental illness.

(iv) 1,100 homeless people living in hostels for the homeless or other such institutions; also including people sleeping rough.

The Clinical Interview Schedule was used to measure 'neurotic psychopathology' (Lewis, Pelosi, et al. 1992). This is a standardized interview, designed to be administered by a trained lay interviewer. The 10,000 adults were asked about the presence of 14 selected symptoms in the past month, and their frequency, severity, and duration in the past week. For psychosis, respondents were screened for reported psychotic behaviour (Bebbington and Nayani 1995), and possible sufferers were followed up with the SCAN (Wing, Babor, et al. 1990). Alcohol and drug dependence were assessed from answers to a self-completion questionnaire.

The findings were broadly similar to those of other community surveys; for instance, about one in seven adults living in private households had some sort of 'neurotic health problem' in the week prior to interview, with women far more likely to suffer from this than men. The four most common neurotic symptoms were fatigue (27%), sleep problems (25%), irritability (22%), and worry (20%). In terms of ICD-10 disorders, the most prevalent in the week prior to interview were Mixed Anxiety and Depressive Disorder (71/1000), and Generalized Anxiety Disorder (30/1000). The overall rate for the whole survey of alcohol dependence was 47/1000 and for drug dependence 22/1000; men were three times more likely than women to have alcohol dependence and twice as likely to be drug dependent, the highest rates being in young men aged 16–24.

7.3 **Across Europe: The European Study of the Epidemiology of Mental Disorders (ESEMeD)**

This was the first European-wide survey of the prevalence of mood and anxiety disorders, and alcohol-related disorders, together with the use of health care services. A modified version of the Composite International Diagnostic Interview (CIDI 3.0) was used, and the study was based upon a sample of 21, 425 non-institutionalized adults selected in Belgium, France, Germany, Italy, the Netherlands, and Spain (representing an overall population of more than 212 million).

Twenty-five percent of participants reported a lifetime presence of any mental disorder, with 11.5% reporting a mental disorder during the past 12 months. The highest rates were found in females, the unmarried, the young, and the unemployed, with frequent co-morbidity. Only 36.8% of those with a mood disorder and 20.6% of those with an anxiety disorder had sought help from health care services; of these, 20.7% received no treatment. Associated levels of disability and reductions in quality of life exceeded levels seen in patients with chronic physical conditions.

7.4 **In seventeen countries worldwide: The World Mental Health Survey of the World Health Organization**

This survey was a remarkable feat of organization and cooperation, and not surprisingly is the largest of its kind ever carried out. The size and complexity of the whole operation required to complete the survey is illustrated by the fact that there are 23 co-authors listed in the above publication. It involved 85,052 subjects in seventeen countries in Africa, Asia, the Americas, Europe, and the Middle East. Lifetime prevalence, projected lifetime risk, and age of onset of DSM-IV disorders were assessed with the WHO Composite International Diagnostic Interview (CIDI). The information from the surveys was subjected to a wide range of sophisticated analyses, and possible sources of both under- and over-reporting are discussed.

To quote just a few results, the estimated lifetime prevalence of having one or more disorder varies from 47.4% in the USA to 12.0% in Nigeria; anxiety disorders were the most prevalent in ten countries, and mood disorders in six. The early onset of many disorders is noted, with many persons waiting for more than ten years before seeking treatment. This highlights the importance of studying whether efforts should be made to ensure earlier access to treatment.

7.5 **Do large-scale surveys of mental disorders have any effect on the provision of mental health services?**

A chief justification for the conduct of epidemiological surveys of mental disorders is often stated as the collection of information that is necessary for the formulation of policy about mental health care and the planning of mental health care. Good estimates of the prevalence and incidence of mental disorders, it is argued, allow the rational allocation of resources. The numbers of people who need mental health care and are not getting it is put forward as an important element in the formulation of policies and in the assignment of priorities for public health action.

These statements ring true, but miss the point. Surveys provide useful but not sufficient arguments for either of the two goals. Mental health needs are not defined by epidemiological surveys alone and policies are formulated using other inputs in addition to epidemiological data.

Mental health needs depend on three determinants: first, how many people have the problem, second, how many of them would accept or demand treatment if it was available, and third, is there an effective intervention that can reduce the severity of the illness or remove it. See Figure 7.1.

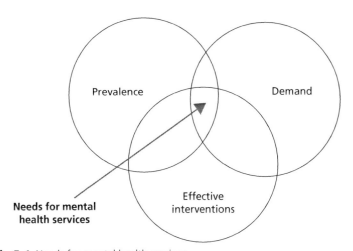

Fig. 7.1 Needs for mental health services.

Thus, needs for mental health services would only be equal to the prevalence of mental disorders, if all the people who have the disease were able to recognize their illness and accept treatment, and if there were an effective treatment that would help all or most of them (delivered in a service or institution that is acceptable to them). In all other instances, mental health needs are less than the prevalence of disorders suggests, although they appear larger if the population's demand is increased. Equally, needs for services can be increased if the population becomes aware of the presence of the disease, can recognize it, and demands care; or if the interventions become very effective, which will make people with the problem for which there is a good (or apparently effective) treatment come forward and ask for help.

The formulation of mental health policies does take the prevalence of mental disorders (or the opinions about the prevalence of mental disorders) into account, but the determining factor is not simply the number of people who have the illness. Four other groups of factors play much more significant roles. These are the perception of the problem, the history of past successes and failures of government policies, the attitudes and aspirations of the health care personnel, and the changes in the context of health care.

The perception of the problem depends on the speed of its development, the feeling of vulnerability of the population (including the politicians), and the impact that the disease has on the individual. AIDS, for example, came out of the blue, grew rapidly, and—while in the beginning mainly striking homosexual men—soon became a menace to whoever was having sex. The disease was lethal and contagious. The first congress concerning AIDS brought together some 15,000 people. There were proposals to create sidatoria in which people with AIDS could be placed, so as to be less of a menace to the population. The policy proposing this was rejected but other policies were adopted, rapidly. Never before was so much money raised so fast as in this case.

Mental disorders are not increasing in numbers very rapidly. Stigma of mental illness makes individuals hide their illness and families deny that any one of their members has it. Mental disorders are not contagious (although the belief that psychiatrists eventually become similar to their patients is held by too many). The mental disorders are not considered curable and the treatments which exist are not considered very effective. Locking up those affected by mental illness is for many the best way to diminish the danger stemming from the unpredictable behaviour that the disease produces. The development of policies about mental health is therefore a slow process (in the period between 1970 and 1990, WHO's insistence made nearly 70% of all countries adopt mental health policies) but their application is sluggish.

The history of past successes and failures of government policies is another factor that determines whether a policy (or a programme) will be adopted, developed, and enforced. Governments fear scandals and many a policy is an answer to public outcries. The policies which are adopted do not necessarily reflect the size of the problem (which might have been established by a prevalence survey) or the evidence about the most effective solutions for it. They provide an answer which will be politically expedient and it is likely that the formulation of a policy will be similar to those that have been effective in this way in the past.

The attitudes and expectations of health service staff are also determinants of health policies. Health personnel find ways to influence policy-making and their reasoning is often not based on the frequency of mental disorders even when they are aware of it, or have been involved in the conduct of epidemiological enquiries. Thus, while staff might be aware of the fact that the placement of patients in the community might improve the quality of life of the patient, they will also consider the inconvenience of visiting patients in their domicile rather than having them on a closed ward in the hospital. They might also argue for policies that will make their work easier, even if that means that fewer people with mental disorders will get treatment: epidemiological assessments of the total numbers of mentally ill people in the community do not seem to have a commanding role in their advice to decision-makers.

Finally, policies about mental health care also depend on the overall socio-economic context in which they are created. Emphasis on cost-effectiveness, increased attention to ethnic differences, high unemployment rates, and numerous other developments in the society influence policies and have a more powerful effect on them than epidemiological data.

In summary, while epidemiology remains an important method of scientific enquiry and might contribute important new knowledge, epidemiological surveys do not have an immediate and powerful impact on mental health policies, or on the organization of services for people with mental illness. The data that surveys produce eventually enter into the consciousness of the general population and of the decision-makers, and will play a role in making policies, but the impact of data is rarely immediate or determinant.

7.6 General conclusions from the results of surveys

If all these surveys carried out in so many countries and cultures are viewed as a whole, two general conclusions can be drawn. First, about the frequency of particular mental disorders, and second, about the effects of these upon the provision of mental health services. In terms of particular mental disorders, it is clear that depressive disorders are the most frequent. The prevalence of depressive disorders in the population is approximately 3–5%; among those contacting general health services, this rises to 5–15% (Ustun and Sartorius 1995). Troublesome states of anxiety are not far behind, together with various forms of distress expressed as physical complaints, but with no identifiable physical illness. The schizophrenic syndromes are found in all cultures, with a lifetime incidence always close to about 1%; these illnesses can often, but not always, lead to severe and long-term social disability, so they are of special importance.

More surprising than any of the information about particular disorders is the universal finding that large proportions of those persons suffering from disorders have never received treatment for these from a psychiatrist. Some of them have contacted general practitioners and other primary health care personnel, and have received treatment (often having been given a diagnosis of a somatic disorder or 'medically unexplained symptoms'). Some have seen traditional practitioners, but many have never sought help from any type of health service. This is the case for countries with comparatively well-developed mental health services just as much as in countries less well placed. This mismatch between having a disorder and getting treatment for it in a country with large numbers of psychiatrists and a variety of services for the mentally ill, was first brought into prominence in the USA by means of the ECA study and the subsequent National Co-morbidity Survey, but it has since been shown to be a universal finding. However, it is not easy to interpret the significance of this finding, since many mental disorders, although troublesome for a time, are self-limiting so do not require treatment. Also, some persons refuse treatment that is offered. In other words, in any community a complicated balance exists between these effects, made even more complicated by the fact that demands for mental health services can often be unrealistic.

Chapter 8

Some problems with research methods used in diagnostic surveys

8.1 Expressed complaints and inferred symptoms

An important problem arises from the nature of the assessment instrument used in a survey as a basis for the diagnoses quoted in the results. The problem is whether expressed complaints, as measured by the DIS and the CIDI, are more relevant and useful than inferred symptoms, as defined and measured by the PSE and SCAN? There is no simple answer to this question.

In the original publications presenting the ECA study, the authors discuss at length the extent to which the ratings on the DIS can be regarded as equivalent to symptoms elicited by a trained clinician. They conclude that the DIS rates 'should be viewed as approximations to rates for selected DSM-III categories' (Robins and Regier 1981). How approximate remains a problem, and the same applies to results from the use of the successor to the DIS, the Composite International Diagnostic Interview (CIDI), discussed later. The debate continues, and anybody planning a large-scale survey should consider carefully which one they prefer to measure in their study.

This important problem arises from the nature of the ratings made during the interview. The trained lay interviewer records the the subject's complaints, which reflect the unpleasantness and suffering of the illness experience; only the subject knows how bad these are. The clinician has been taught to regard some, but not all, of these complaints as symptoms that indicate the presence of a treatable disorder, so these will be selected and given precedence by the clinician in conceptualizing what is wrong, and deciding whether there is a need for treatment. Until there is some improvement in understanding and measuring the abnormal processes that underlie both the symptoms and the complaints, the problem as to which should be the best basis for action will remain. Another problem is that neither complaints nor symptoms correlate as well as might be expected with demand for treatment, as noted in Section 7.5. The demand for treatment is also influenced by the personality characteristics of the patient, the presence of other illnesses, and the reputation of the psychiatrist and the psychiatric service.

8.2 Comparison of complaints and symptoms in field studies

8.2.1 Comparison of the DIS and the PSE

The organizers of the ECA studies were, of course, aware of this problem, and carried out some studies in which selected survey subjects were interviewed twice, once by a lay interviewer using the DIS and then shortly afterwards by a psychiatrist using a PSE-type interview schedule (Anthony, Folstein, Romanoski, et al. 1985; Helzer, Robins, McEvoy, et al. 1985).

Figures 8.1 and 8.2 show the results of one of the comparison studies carried out by Anthony et al. (1985). This, and other published papers from the study, contain many such tables, but this example has been selected because it illustrates several points of special interest. The comparison study was carried out on a selected sub-sample of 810 Baltimore subjects. After the ordinary DIS interview by a lay interviewer, the subject was interviewed again by a psychiatrist using a clinical reassessment (CR). This was a semi-structured PSE-style interview (that is, using extra probe questions when the interviewer wished, and always trying to get a description of a recent example from the subject of an occasion when the symptom in question was experienced). The psychiatrist did not know the results of the first interview, and more than half of the repeat interviews were carried out within two weeks of the first interview. The table is of the one-month prevalence of a number of selected DSM-III diagnoses in the 810 subjects. Figure 8.1 shows the results expressed as group rates.

The psychiatrist found roughly twice as many persons as the lay interviewer with Phobic Disorder, and similarly for alcohol misuse. In contrast, the lay interviewer found about twice as many subjects with Major Depressive Disorder than the psychiatrist. For schizophrenia, the rates were much closer: 0.7% for the lay interviewer compared to 0.5% for the psychiatrist. However, a cross tabulation, as in Figure 8.2, shows how these rates originate. The cross-tabulation of the 33 subjects diagnosed as having schizophrenia by either one of the interviewers shows that there was agreement in only three subjects out of the 33.

This example illustrates how group rates can conceal important individual differences due to the methods used, and why many psychiatrists are uneasy about the meaning of survey results derived from use of the DIS.

DSM-Diagnoses	Lay DIS	Psychiatrist (CR)
Phobic Disorder	11.2	21.3
Alchohol Mis-use	3.6	6.9
Major Depression	2.3	1.1
Obsessive Compulsive	1.3	0.3
Panic Disorder	0.8	0.1
Schiziophrenia	0.7	0.5

Fig. 8.1 Selected DSM-III diagnoses. Lay DIS vs psychiatrist (CR). One month prevalence rates n = 180 (sub-sample). > 50% repeated within two weeks. Data from Anthony et al. (1985).

		Psychiatrist (CR) +	Psychiatrist (CR) −	
Lay Interviewer (DIS)	+	3	16	19
Lay Interviewer (DIS)	−	11	780	791
		14	796	810

Fig. 8.2 DSM-III diagnosis of schizophrenia. Cross-tabulation of 33 individuals. Rates use 14 and 19, but there was agreement on only 3 persons out of 14 and 19 = 33. Data from Anthony et al. (1985).

Unfortunately, in the absence of any other independent objective measurements, it is not possible to say whether the complaints or the symptoms should be preferred as a basis for action. It is to be expected that psychiatrists will prefer to regard the symptoms as having more meaning than the complaints, but social workers and clinical psychologists are likely to give at least as much importance to the complaints.

8.2.2 Comparison of SCAN and CIDI

Similar comparison studies were done in the UK Survey of Psychiatric Morbidity carried out in 1993 (Melzer, Gill, et al. 1995). A special additional study was carried out in which some subjects were interviewed using the successors to the DIS and the PSE, namely the Composite International Diagnostic Interview (CIDI) and the Schedules for Clinical Assessment in Neuropsychiatry (SCAN) (Brugha et al. 2001). Figure 8.3 shows the SCAN and CIDI results for 172 selected subjects interviewed at home, assessed as having any depressive episode or disorder (with a maximum of 14 days between interviews).

In this example, the CIDI interview with a lay interviewer clearly picks out many more subjects than the SCAN interview conducted by a psychiatrist but again, agreement on individuals is limited to only three subjects. The report of this study contains a detailed discussion of this whole problem.

It is obvious that the interviews are measuring different things, but how best to use these results remains unclear. Follow-up studies to discover which

		Psychiatrist Scan		
		+	−	
Lay Interviewer CIDI	+	3	22	25
	−	3	144	147
		6	166	172

Fig. 8.3 Are expressed complaints (CIDI) equivalent to inferred symptoms (SCAN)? 172 subjects at home (selected). Any depressive episode or disorder. Maximum of 14 days between interviews. Data from Brugha et al. (2001).

of the two ratings (i.e. complaints or symptoms) is most closely correlated with disability, the seeking of treatment, and the response to treatment have yet to be done.

Further critical discussion of the DIS ratings has come from research centres outside the USA, notably from Australia. P. Burvill in Perth commented upon a variety of the problems noted above (Burvill 1987), and G. Parker in Sydney provided a detailed and energetic criticism of the lifetime prevalence estimates, particularly of the depressive disorders (Parker 1987). Nevertheless, the attractiveness of being able to do large-scale mental health surveys without using expensive psychiatrists has meant that the CIDI has wide and continued usage.

8.3 The use of short rather than lengthy rating scales

In all interviewing schedules, each question is followed by a rating scale which gives the interviewer options for recording the presence or absence of whatever is being asked about, and if present, the severity. This often takes the form of 0 = absent, 1 = mild, and 2 = severe (with further definition of what these terms mean). But some rating scales are more ambitious and contain ratings for three or even more degrees of severity. Such a degree of exactness can seem tempting to those who are designing an investigation, but it brings with it some problems of data analysis which are likely to be insoluble. First, the inter-rater reliability of fine rating divisions will need to be tested (and will usually be found to be very low), and second, when the results are examined during the preliminary stages of data analysis, it is likely that the number of ratings of each separate degree of severity will be very uneven, in that some will have been used frequently and some hardly at all. The statistical advisor to the study will then point out that condensation of the fine degrees of severity into a simpler scale (of probably two or at the most three points) will have to be done before sensible use can be made of the data. In other words, a simpler rating scale may as well have been used in the first place, and the task of the interviewer would have been easier. (Anybody designing a survey is strongly advised to involve a statistical advisor in the design of rating schedules from the start of planning.)[1]

8.4 Differences between 'bottom-up' and 'top-down' interviewing schedules

In the world of project planning and business management techniques, the concepts of 'bottom-up' and 'top-down' are well known. In the 'up' approach, there is a move from detailed small-scale ideas and activities towards larger concepts, and in the 'down' approach there is the opposite movement from broad ideas and activities to their more detailed components. The same applies to 'up' or 'down' when used to describe an interviewing schedule, with refererence to the set of ideas upon which the schedule was originally based. The simplest example is the DIS, which is a 'down' schedule, designed to detect the symptoms of a selection of the most common and important disorders in DSM-III to be rated for the ECA studies. The criteria for each disorder are rephrased as questions, and the subject's reply is recorded by the interviewer choosing one of several options provided in the schedule. The schedule contains only questions derived from the lists of criteria, plus some questions designed to eliminate false positives due to the presence of physical illness or side-effects of medication. The interviewer does not ask any other questions about frequency, severity, or the general circumstances to do with the occuurence of possible syptoms. The intensive training course for the DIS is based upon these principles, which also apply to the the CIDI, successor to the DIS.

Since 'top-down' schedules are derived from a previously existing document, any change in that document means that the interviewing schedule must be changed to reflect this. Thus, any change in the DSM classification has to be followed by a change in the interviewing schedule, in addition to changes in any computer programs used to analyse the ratings.

In contrast, the content of an 'up' schedule, such as the PSE and SCAN, is not limited to items that might contribute to a disorder. It is determined by the wider purpose of the schedule, which is to provide ratings that will give a complete description of all the symptoms and complaints of the subject, needed to allow a full description of the subject's clinical state. Questions about diagnostic symptoms are, of course, prominent in the schedule, but other questions cover potentially troublesome but non-diagnostic symptoms (such as muscular tension and excessive worrying). In addition, the interviewer is encouraged to ask, if thought suitable, additional questions not provided in the written schedule, such as 'What was it like?', 'Please tell me more', 'Can you give me an example?', that might clarify whether the symptom in question was definitely present or not, to what degree, and the amount of distress it has caused. This difference is why the training period for the CIDI can be shorter that that for the SCAN, so long as the CIDI interviewer is already familiar with the general idea of interviewing. For successful use of the SCAN, it is assumed that the interviewer also needs to have had some sort of clinical experience gained from contact with medical, psychological, or psychiatric patients, before going through the special training for the SCAN. Since the content of PSE and SCAN is comprehensive and not tied to any particular classification, revision of the ICD classification needs to be followed only by changes in the associated computer programs, and not by changes in the interview schedules.

Note

1 Here is some advice which I have never known to be followed exactly, even by myself. But it is eminently sensible, and acts as an ideal to be aimed at. The researchers who are going to be responsible for the data analysis and publication of the results of a survey should work out, before the survey begins, the layout of the tables which will be used to present the major findings. In other words, a set of dummy tables with the columns and rows specified in detail, but with empty cells, should be prepared. These tables, together with the interview/rating schedules which will be used in the survey, should then be discussed with the statistical advisor before the data collection begins. JEC.

Chapter 9

Translation and use of interviewing schedules for use in more than one language and culture

9.1 Equivalence and authenticity

The awareness of the need to pay attention to the possibility of comparing psychiatric symptoms in different cultural settings began to grow after the Second World War—which contributed to the possibility of international and collaborative research—partly in parallel to the opposition to the view that behaviour can only be measured in its own culture. Berry (1969) has contributed to the resolution of that problem, by proposing that comparisons of behaviour in different cultures can be made, if it can be shown that the behavioural phenomena are functionally equivalent. Functional equivalence was postulated to be present when the behaviours to be compared are responses to the same stimulus or problem; in such instances the culture-specific descriptions of the behaviours can be used to develop a framework in which the behaviours can be compared. If this position is accepted, then cross-cultural comparisons of behaviour are possible and valid.

Another concept proposed in the late 1970s is that of authenticity (Pareek and Rao 1980). Authenticity refers to the capacity of an interviewer to get genuine answers from the respondent. It depends on four sets of factors; those related to the interviewer (e.g. the interviewer's profession), those related to the respondent (e.g. the previous experience of the respondent), those specific to the setting in which the interview takes place (e.g. in a hospital or at home), and those related to the culture in which the interview takes place (e.g. norms of courtesy).

Both concepts—the authenticity and the 'legitimacy' of cross-cultural comparisons—are of direct relevance to the work comparing the forms, and course of mental disorders, in different cultures. The third element that needs to be considered, when attempting to compare psychiatric phenomena in different cultures, is that of the language equivalence of the instruments used in the examination of the mental states of people living in different cultures.

The importance of achieving equivalence of instruments used in different languages varies with the level of standardization of the instruments. Fully standardized instruments do not allow the interviewer to help the respondent to answer questions and require full equivalence of the instruments. The same is true of instruments which the respondents are expected to fill in themselves. Semi-standardized instruments in which the interviewer is trained in the use of the instrument and formulates the questions to the respondent in a manner that is culturally appropriate require less work on equivalence but considerably more work on the training of the interviewers. The same is true for free clinical interviews which are carried out by well-trained interviewers aiming to make a diagnosis or develop a summary of the patients' condition.

The disadvantage of the fully standardized instruments is that they do not resemble the normal conversations between the respondents and the interviewers, which can be upsetting for the respondents and lead them to produce random, meaningless, or misleading answers to questions that they do not understand or dislike. The disadvantage of the free interviews is that they may be widely different in coverage and neglect important aspects of the respondents' condition. The semi-standardized instruments are a happy compromise, in that they force the well-trained interviewers to get answers to all the questions contained in the interview, but allow them to use culturally appropriate ways of phrasing the question (or questions that they need to add) so as to obtain the information which will allow them to rate the presence or absence of the phenomena covered by the instrument.

Regardless of the type of instrument—fully, partially, or non-standardized—it will be necessary to establish its equivalence in the languages in which it will be used. There are three types of equivalence, all of importance for the validity of the information obtained by the use of the instrument: the semantic equivalence, the conceptual equivalence, and the technical equivalence.

The semantic equivalence is achieved when the words in the source language and the target language (into which the question in an instrument is being translated) have corresponding denotations and connotations. The denotation of a word is its dictionary definition: thus, an apple is defined as a fruit with a specific shape, taste, season of ripening, and so on. The connotation of the word refers to the emotional content of a word; thus in relation to the apple, it might refer to its shape being attractive or its taste delicious. The connotations of words can be examined using instruments such as Osgood's semantic differential which requires the respondent to place the word which is being examined on a series of visual analogue scales that have ends defined in terms such as 'beautiful' and 'ugly'. Semantic equivalence can also be assessed by the overlap of the semantic spheres of words: semantic spheres are defined by all the synonyms that a word has: thus, by this method, two words are semantically equivalent if they, as well as most of their synonyms, are matching.(Wing, Sartorius, and Ustun 1998). The conceptual equivalence refers to the position and significance of a word in the theoretical system to which it belongs. Thus, 'loss of face' might be of such importance in one culture that it would lead to suicide, while in another culture it is no more than an aggravation without much significance: in this instance, the 'loss of face' should be avoided as a descriptor or example in the instrument that will be used in a comparative study of the two cultures concerned.

Technical equivalence refers to the way in which the items should be formulated to convey the same meaning. Thus, for example, in some languages comparisons are not used to explain or measure a meaning: in such an instance, questions such as, 'Do you feel as bad as if you had lost a lot of money?' will not be useful because the answer will invariably be, 'I did not lose any money' or, 'Why would you like to know about my loss of money?'

The assessment of the level of equivalence achieved by a translation is best preceded by the examination of the instrument by a group of persons who are bilingual and know the culture in which the instruments will be used. The bilingual group will produce an overall judgement about the usability of the instrument in the two languages and cultures. Once this is done, the instrument can be translated from the original to the target language. At this point, it is important to decide whether the instrument will be fully standardized (i.e. whether all the questions will be presented to the respondents in the same way by an interviewer who is not allowed to add any comments or explanations), or semi-standardized. Semi-standardized instruments are used by skilful, well-trained interviewers who understand the intent of each question, and conduct the interview in a culture-appropriate manner to obtain an answer to the question. Fully standardized instruments should be back-translated from the target to the source language, and the two originals and the back-translation compared. The process of back-translation should be repeated until the back-translation and the original are matching (the reiterative back-translation method). The members of the bilingual group should then discuss the translated version with monolingual users of the instrument to explore whether the questions make sense and can be understood by the interviewers.

For semi-standardized instruments, the key to equivalence is intensive training of the interviewers. The instruments do not have to be fully back-translated. It is usually sufficient to carry out 'target checks' of questions that are addressing sensitive matters. The discussion of the bilingual group members and the monolingual group of interviewers should, however, take place.

9.2 Guidelines for schedules to be used in more than one language

When composing instruments that are likely to be used in more than one language, the following should be kept in mind:

- Restrict each item to one topic or enquiry
  - Use short sentences
  - Use active rather than passive voice
  - Use nouns rather than pronouns
  - Avoid metaphors
  - Avoid colloquial expressions
  - Avoid conditional expressions
  - Avoid the verbs 'would' and 'could'
  - Avoid possessive forms
  - Avoid imprecise words such as 'probably'
  - Avoid sentences containing alternatives answers to a question

Studies that have been carried out under the auspices of the World Health Organization in the two decades from 1970–1990 demonstrated that semi-standardized instruments used by carefully trained interviewers, who have an opportunity to discuss the interview and its application, are by far the most efficient way of arriving at the equivalence of the questionnaires and valid answers about the respondents' condition. Financial constraints may prevent the joint training of interviewers, and it might be necessary to resort to cheaper ways of making the interviewers accept and interiorize the same understanding of the examination (e.g. videotaped interviews with expert commentaries). Every effort should be made to train the interviewers in collaborative studies involving subjects in different cultures, in the same place, and at the same time.

9.3 Culture-specific disorders

Are there any culture-specific disorders whose equivalents cannot be found in other cultures? This issue has often been debated in the past, and sets a special problem for classifications. In the hope of stimulating research into the possibility of finding disorders that exist in some cultures but not in others, a special section on 'culture-specific' disorders was added as an appendix to the diagnostic criteria for research (DCR-10) developed for ICD-10 (WHO 1993). As noted in the introduction to this appendix, 'These syndromes have also been referred to as culture-bound or culture-reactive, and as ethnic or exotic psychoses. Some are rare and some may be comparatively common; many are acute and transient, which makes their systematic study particularly difficult'. There is also a 'Glossary of culture-bound syndromes' in Appendix I of DSM-IV-TR (APA 2000).

Over the last few decades, it seems that the importance of this debate has lessened. The possible reasons for this include first, that the increase in psychiatric services across the world has shown that any difference between disorders in different cultures is in prevalence rather than existence. Second, differences in levels of education in the persons affected and in the nature of the services available have an effect upon how various forms of distress are expressed, but the basic symptoms causing the distress are those of disorders already in the classification.

Even if some culture-specific disorders did exist in the past, there are some recent influences which might well blur the distinction between them and disorders already established in the classifications. For instance, the large migrations of people from one culture to another that have occurred in the last hundred years or so have led to a mixing of cultural ways of expressing distress, thus obscuring any culturally specific syndromes that might have existed. In addition, new and effective methods of treatment for a wide variety of symptoms have become increasingly widespread; doctors are therefore more likely to make diagnoses of disorders already in the classification, if the symptoms are similar to those of the patient. There is usually a praiseworthy modern emphasis on cultural influences when assessing a patient, but this consists of taking the cultural background of patients into consideration when trying to understand the background of the development and treatment of more familiar disorders already in the classifications. However, none of these points can be regarded as positive evidence that culture-specific disorders do not exist, and further epidemiologically based research would be well worthwhile.

Chapter 10

Towards international agreement on classification

10.1 The development of ICD-9

ICD-9, published by WHO in 1978, was to some extent a holding operation. The separate publication of the glossary to ICD-8 had been widely welcomed, as had many changes in all the other non-psychiatric chapters of the rest of the ICD. Acceptance and adaptation of any changes that might be suggested for ICD-9 would need some time in a worldwide context, so a conservative approach to ICD-9 was announced by the ICD office in Geneva. The compilers of all the chapters of ICD-9 and their advisors were asked to leave any radical changes that might be under consideration until ICD-10 was due. There had already been some discussion among the WHO staff and their advisors about the possibility of including lists of diagnostic criteria in Chapter V of ICD-9, alongside the narrative clinical descriptions, but this overall conservative policy for the whole of ICD-9 meant that such a change had to postponed for a few years until ICD-10. Nevertheless, some improvements were made in ICD-9, the most important being an expansion of those categories dealing with disorders of childhood and adolescence, and the specification of adjustment and stress reactions.

10.2 The Joint Project: Collaboration between the World Health Organization and the National Institute of Mental Health of the USA

In the late 1970s, Gerald Klerman, then Director of the National Institute of Alcohol, Drug Abuse, and Mental Health Agency of the USA, expressed keen interest in the collaborative development of psychiatric assessment instruments and in the revisions of the classification of mental disorders. His interest found expression in the provision of a grant to the Division of Mental Health of the World Health Organization, for work on these subjects. From the start, the basic strategy of the Project was to recognize the essentially international nature of progress in many aspects of mental health work, particularly for classification and diagnosis, and to minimize the eventual differences between Chapter V of ICD-10 and DSM-IV. The Project, developed in collaboration between the two organizations, was undoubtedly the largest international effort in this field.

The work of the Project was in three phases. First, in preparation for a major conference, nine scientific groups prepared review papers that formed the background document for the conference. Second, the conference was held in Copenhagen in 1982, attended by some 200 psychiatrists (Cooper 1982b). The third stage was planned as an ongoing and open-ended programme of collaborative field studies based upon the objectives and priorities that would be identified by the conference.

Proposals for the revision of the 10th Revision of the WHO International Classification of Diseases were central activities in this programme, together with instruments for obtaining information that is necessary for the study and diagnosis of mental disorders. The Combined International Diagnostic Instrument (CIDI) was developed from the Diagnostic Interview Schedule (Robins, Wing, Wittchen, et al. 1988), and the Schedule for the Clinical Assessment in Neuropsychiatry (SCAN) was produced with the PSE-10 as its core feature (Wing et al. 1990). The development of both of these consisted of adding sufficient items to cover all the disorders (except personality disorders) present in ICD-10 and DSM-IV, and the writing of computer programs so that diagnoses from both ICD-10 and DSM-IV could be derived from either interview. To arrive at a diagnosis of one of the personality disorders requires a different interviewing technique, and a set of items of a different style. To cope with these differences, the International Personality Disorder Examination (IPDE) was produced under the guidance of Loranger (Loranger, Sartorius, et al. 1994). These instruments have now been widely used in many countries.

10.3 The development of ICD-10 Chapter V

This took about 10 years, from 1982 to 1992. An account of the many facets of this programme can be found in Supplement 1 to Volume 152 of the British Journal of Psychiatry; (Jablensky, Sartorius, et al. 1983; Sartorius et al. 1988), but some of the main points are noted here. In the background of the many activities involved was the theme of the 1982 Copenhagen conference; that it would be to everybody's benefit if major dissimilarities and incompatibilities between ICD-10 and DSM-IV could be avoided.

As part of the overall ICD system, Chapter V has to be acceptable and understandable to psychiatrists in countries with differing degrees of development of medical education and mental health services. This means that every revision of the ICD must be based upon widespread consultations. Established recent advances in knowledge need to be included, but the enthusiastic recommendations and advice of the experts of the day at the forefront of research units in comparatively wealthy countries have to be balanced with a generally conservative approach to changes. An early decision was made to follow a strategy of 'different versions for different purposes', and priority was given to development of the full clinical version, called 'Clinical Descriptions and Diagnostic Guidelines' (CDDG).

The process was started in Geneva in 1982; more than 50 individual experts in a wide variety of countries were asked by Jablensky and Sartorius to provide first drafts for the main sections. This input was then edited and put together into one document, and circulated to a further 200 experts in 1983 and 1984, for further development and comments. The World Psychiatric Association then gave invaluable help by circulating a second draft to all its member societies and associations, resulting in another set of comments and criticisms. The resulting draft then underwent extensive field trials in 1987 and 1988 (Burke 1988; Sartorius et al. 1993) using 112 Field Trial Centres in 39 countries, coordinated by twelve Field Trial Coordinating Centres. Translation of the documents required for the field trials into six languages (French, German, Spanish, Arabic, Chinese, and Japanese) was undertaken by the directors of the Field Trial Coordinating Centres.

One of the final activities of the Joint Project was to support the attendance of several of the WHO advisors to ICD-10 at a series of four meetings between 1988 and 1992, at which the leaders of the some of the DSM-IV Task Forces were preparing the final drafts of DSM-IV. Whenever possible, the same concepts, diagnostic terms, and descriptions were agreed for use in both the classifications, and the reasons for those differences that remained were clarified. The result is that there are surprisingly few differences of any importance between the final versions of the two classifications; those remaining are largely the result of the different audiences that the classifications serve (Regier, Kaelber, et al. 1994). WHO must produce a common language for a diverse set of users, but the DSM-IV is more influenced by the clinical and financial priorities of the American Psychiatric Association. More detailed comments on this issue can be found in Appendix D of the full version of DSM-IV, and in Cooper (1995).

10.4 The family of documents of ICD-10 Chapter V

Based directly on the CDDG, additional documents were then prepared. First, a shorter version of the clinical descriptions was needed to go into the main volume of ICD-10, containing all 21 chapters, alongside the nomenclature and code numbers (see Appendix 5.) Second, a set of Diagnostic Criteria for Research (DCR-10, WHO 1993) was derived from the CDDG. Included as appendix to the DCR-10 is a list and glossary of the so-called 'culture-specific' disorders, in the hope of encouraging research into their epidemiology and defining characteristics. Third, a short and simple version for use in primary care (ICD-10-PHC) was developed. This is of great potential importance globally, since the majority of the world's population receives its psychiatric care in the setting of primary care services (Ustun and Satorius 1995). The ICD-10-PHC contains only the 24 disorders most frequently seen in primary care, and is presented quite differently from the other versions (WHO 1996). Brief notes about presentation and main diagnostic features are given, plus information for patient and family, counselling techniques, and indications for drug therapy and specialist referral. There is also a very brief version of the classification containing only six categories, for use by primary care workers who have only minimal qualifications.

A multiaxial classification for use in child and adolescent psychiatry was also produced (WHO 1966); this is discussed in Chapter 16.

Chapter 11

Communication between health care professions

11.1 Different versions for different purposes

The idea of different versions of the same classification for different users has been around in the international psychiatric literature since the 1930s (see Lewis 1938) but, although clearly sensible, it was not put into practice by compilers of classifications until the 1990s when WHO did this for ICD-10. Foremost among the reasons for this is the lack of firm evidence that most psychiatric disorders can be regarded as distinct 'nosological entities', that is, easily definable and separated from each other by such things as their pathogenesis, course, response to treatment, and outcome (Jablensky 2012).

Up to now, the consequence of the fact that psychiatry is not dealing with easily definable nosological entities has been the development of different classifications for different purposes and by different groups, but these classifications are not compatible with each other. For instance, general practitioners have a classification of mental disorders organized in a manner that corresponds to what they see in their patients and what makes them take one or another line of action. The World Association of National Colleges, Academies, and Academic Associations of General Practitioners/Family Physicians (WONCA) produced such a classification including mental disorders, and recommended it to its members (WONCA 1986). Insurance companies naturally have focussed on the amount of impairment and the severity of the disability that a particular condition might cause, and a number of companies have created such classifications. Researchers have set quite strict criteria for inclusion of conditions or syndromes into categories that maximize the probability that the persons whom they study do not differ in their symptoms or other characteristics. Nurses have developed classifications that they feel are useful in their work, and specialists in rehabilitation have created classifications that make sense from the point of view of rehabilitative practice.

There are two main problems with this state of affairs. The first is that the classifications which have been produced are not of equal quality. Some of them are not comprehensive and some have no operational or other criteria which would facilitate the placement of conditions into categories. Some are not regularly updated; others are so complicated that their use is limited. The second problem is that the existing classifications are not compatible with each other; this makes communication difficult or impossible between those who use the classifications.

The first of these two problems could be at least mitigated by accompanying the classifications with a set of explanations, rules, and guidance for use, and by making the acceptance of the classifications dependent on their application. A great deal of cooperation and agreement between the compilers and users of the classifications is needed for this approach to be successful. The second problem of incompatibility is much more serious, but there are two ways of dealing with it. First, a 'master classification' could be produced, and then a way found to force all those who deal with conditions that are being classified to use that classification. This might be possible if there was only one profession that deals with a particular set of health conditions, and if all of the members of that profession were to be educated in the same way about the use of the classification. This strategy faces difficulties when health workers from different countries (educated in different ways) and of different professions are expected to use such a classification. The second solution is to produce a 'master' classification and then several versions of it for specific purposes—ensuring, however, that they are translatable back to the master classification. This strategy has to overcome the problem that the users of a classification designed for a particular profession are usually reluctant to accept the inevitable, although minor, constraints of translatability.

Following the latter strategy, the WHO, as part of their Joint Project with the NIMH of the USA (see Section 10.2) produced three versions of the 'master classification' of mental and behavioural disorders that is contained along with the other chapters in the main ICD-10 volume (22 in all, see Appendix 5). As described in Section 10.4, these comprise one for clinical use by practising psychiatrists, one for research purposes, and one for use in primary health care settings. Provision of useful documents, however, does not by itself ensure that they will be widely used. The clinical version, the Clinical Descriptions and Diagnostic Guidelines (CDDG), has been well accepted, translated into many languages, and is used by psychiatrists in many countries in their daily practice. The research version, Diagnostic Criteria for Research (DCR-10), is less well known and less often used, although it is well-structured and does not differ much from the criteria of the DSM. One of the reasons for this lack of use is that the editors of some psychiatric journals refuse to take papers in which the subjects were diagnosed using the DCR-10, preferring those papers that rely on the DSM. More important in this respect, however, is the fact that the World Health Organization has been far less effective in promoting the use of its classifications than the American Psychiatric Association.

The ICD-10 Chapter V Primary Care Version, entitled *WHO Diagnostic and Management Guidelines for Mental Disorders in Primary Care* (WHO ICD-10-PHC 1996) has been used in a number of settings, often by psychiatrists who find that it serves well to classify the large majority of cases they have seen.

The latest development in this complicated situation is that, with both ICD-11 and DSM-5 in mind, the APA DSM-5 Task Force and the WHO Advisory Group on the Classification of Mental Disorders have been charged with the production of a classification that will be:

1. useful in both primary care and specialist psychiatry

2. suitable for billing for service

3. suitable for the production of national statistics about mental disorders for public health purposes, and

4. serve as an internationally useful common language for researchers who are trying to ensure that their investigations deal with clearly defined homogenous groups of patients.

While doing this, they have to take into account opinions of psychiatrists and other mental health personnel that are far from being unanimous, and reflect practice in different settings and cultures. In other words, they have been set a formidable task, and it is clear that the policy of different versions for different purposes does not appeal to those in charge of the current revision processes.

11.2 The importance of labels

The labels of conditions that are considered to be in the domain of psychiatry, regardless of whether they refer to nosological entities or to ill-defined syndromes, are not only parts of the language of communication among psychiatrists and other health professionals. They also have other functions which are important, but often given insufficient attention (see Chapter 17 for wider effects of classifications). Labels given to diseases are often in danger of becoming labels for persons who have the disease, and this may change their lives. The stigma attached to some disorders can be particularly grave; thus persons with schizophrenia will soon, in the language of doctors and the general public, become 'schizophrenics'. This is likely to ruin their chances for employment, for decent housing, or for the creation of a family.

In view of this type of problem some psychiatrists in Japan, aware of the particularly grave consequences in that country of using the label, recently decided to abandon the Japanese name for schizophrenia and to replace it by another term, accompanied by a different description of the disorder (Sato 2006). An immediate consequence of this change was that the relationship of doctors and their patients changed. Psychiatrists reported that the change of the label made it much easier to convey the diagnosis to the patient and to agree with them on the process of their treatment.

In many countries, the stigma attached to mental illness is also shared by mental health workers. The psychiatrists in particular may be regarded by the general public and even by their medical colleagues as being somewhat similar to their patients and therefore peculiar.[1]

Jablensky (2012) has also drawn attention to the important distinction between validity and utility. The latter does not refer only to the practising psychiatrist and his decision about the most appropriate treatment; there is also utility for public health purposes (e.g. for decisions about the priorities and funding for mental health programmes based on epidemiological studies), utility of the labels that affect the public image of psychiatry and psychiatrists, utility for the organization of training about mental disorders in schools of health personnel, utility for research purposes, and the utility for the management of mentally ill people in primary and other forms of general health care. In all of these instances there would be much benefit for all if we knew that we were dealing with nosological entities, but the issue of utility for different purposes remains just as important, even though this is not yet possible.

The consequence of the uncertainty about the nosological status of conditions which are the domain of psychiatry is that we shall have to live with a variety of classifications, each serving the needs of a particular profession or a particular purpose. For the time being our efforts should be directed to both the search for psychiatric nosological entities (which would allow the production of a reference classification) and to maintaining the translatability of the different classifications into each other. Horses for courses, or, in other words, different classifications for different purposes translatable into each other. This seems to be, for the time being, the least unsatisfactory pathway for psychiatry to follow.

Note

1 When I was a medical student, one of my senior psychiatric teachers surprised me by remarking that if I took up psychiatry, I would find that one of the biggest obstacles to the development of psychiatry and psychiatric services would be the rest of the medical profession. Looking back over the years, I can see that he was right. JEC.

Chapter 12

Understanding classification

12.1 Classification as part of taxonomy: basic rules and definition of terms

What is classification in the strict sense? As already noted, in everyday language to classify things is to arrange them in groups that have some characteristics in common. But there is a more formal use of the term 'classification', as part of the discipline of *taxonomy*. This has its own terms and statistical techniques that can be applied to any field of knowledge that is supported by extensive and reliable data. To arrive at a taxonomically correct classification, it is necessary to go through several stages. First, it is necessary to use an agreed set of names, so that each object being classified (in this case psychiatric disorders) will have only one name. This set of names is called a *nomenclature*. It is also an advantage to state from the onset the main purpose of the nomenclature and classification that is being constructed. In practice, most classifications get used for a variety of purposes, but to have a main purpose clearly stated makes it easier for users to understand its structure, and is a help to those who are constructing it. It is easy to say (and theoretically correct) that the purpose of a classification should be stated clearly from the start, and that this will determine the nature of the criteria used to define the objects and the taxons. But in practice, there are often problems because most classifications get used for several different purposes, for some of which they were not designed.[a]

A nomenclature should also begin with an introductory statement and description (and, if possible, a definition), that indicates the nature of the objects in the nomenclature (such as dogs, birds, diseases of the chest, edible vegetables, etc.). The next step is to agree on a description of the main characteristics of each named object. The collection of all these descriptions together can then be called a *glossary*. The final stage is to refine the descriptions so that they contain a central part that is a *definition*.

---

[a] Those who construct classifications have much in common with lexicographers. Of these, Dr Johnson remarked, 'Every other author may aspire to praise. The lexicographer can only hope to escape reproach.'

A definition contains only a list of properties that are unique to the object that is being defined; that is, they are not possessed by any other object in the nomenclature.

If all these stages are completed, then it is clear what the object being defined is, and also what it is not. The definitions of all the objects in the classification can then be said to be mutually exclusive and jointly exhaustive (a phrase much loved by optimistic classifiers). This means that: (a) every object in the nomenclature is defined so that it cannot be confused with anything else, although it has the features that define the taxon in which it is placed; (b) all the objects that should be in the classification have been included; and (c) each object has only one place.

The above steps indicate how to arrive at a group of objects that have obvious and important similarities. Technically this is called a 'taxon'. For psychiatric disorders as currently recognized, a nomenclature and a glossary can certainly be achieved, but with the proviso that the somewhat imprecise definition of disorder means that opinions on which clinical states should be included in the nomenclature may vary from one clinician to another. In other words, if there is a wish to regard any group of disorders being studied as a taxon, it will have imprecise boundaries.[1]

With this limitation of imprecise boundaries, there is no doubt that most common psychiatric disorders can be grouped into a useful series of taxons, such as depressive disorders, anxiety disorders, delusional disorders, and others. Unfortunately, these psychiatric taxons also have another weakness, in that they can be identified only by descriptions (often subjective), and not by more precise measurements. So the taxonomic quality of both the ICD-10 Chapter V and DSM-IV is not high. The arrangement of sets of taxons into a *taxonomic hierarchy* is discussed in the next section.

12.2 Successful classifications in the biological and physical sciences

12.2.1 The classification of animals

If we examine a very useful classification, such as the biological classification of animals, we see first that the rough equivalent of the set of taxons of psychiatric disorders is the set of taxons of animal species (a species is a group of animals that, in natural surroundings, breeds exclusively within the group). Dogs, cats, bears, horses, and cows are all examples of species. For the biological classification, other possibilities of grouping animals then become evident because of the large additional amount of different types of information and measurements that are available about animals. The taxons of the different species can themselves easily be arranged in groups by means of other properties that are shared by all the animals in several taxons. For instance cats, dogs, and bears are well-defined, separate taxons, and they also are all carnivorous and have claws. In contrast, cows, horses, sheep, and goats are all vegetarians and have hooves. So groups of taxons can be formed, in this case called 'orders', of *carnivores* and *herbivores*. A further even larger group, or class, including both herbivores and carnivores, can be formed of those animals with *mammalian* characteristics (such as mammary glands for suckling young, hair, and sweat glands).

In this way, the animal kingdom can be seen to fall into several layers or levels of taxons and the whole classification of animals is said to form a hierarchy[2] or set of levels. This type of arrangement, called a *taxonomic hierarchy* was first suggested for both plants and animals by Carl Linnaeus, a Swedish biologist, in 1735, using only the descriptive information then available. When Darwinian evolution was described many years later, it became clear that this layered classification, although still based only upon simple descriptive information, also illustrated how evolution has resulted in groups of animals descended from common ancestors. This is most easily seen for animals. More recently, DNA analysis and other modern methods of description, measurement, and analysis have confirmed the usefulness and basic correctness of the taxonomic hierarchy model.

The lesson to be learned from this is that what started out with only simple descriptions of physical appearance and behaviour, as collected by Linnaeus and his contemporaries, has turned out to reflect quite fundamental underlying relationships (at that time unknown) due to the process of evolution. For psychiatric disorders at the present time, there is nothing obvious that might allow the formation of higher layers of taxons that could be the start of a reasonably comprehensive hierarchical classification.[b]

The main deficiency is the lack of objective measurements that could be added to the clinical descriptions now used to identify disorders.[1]

Nevertheless, the search for new measurements and techniques should continue, in the hope of identifying and measuring new mechanisms and processes that underlie the symptoms and behaviours upon which we currently rely. This is not for want of trying, for over the last few decades a very wide range of physiological and biochemical measurements have been applied to patients with psychiatric disorders. Unfortunately, none has been found to be sufficiently specific to any individual clinical disorder or to be usable as a reliable indicator of its presence or absence in individual patients.

---

[b] The same problem of definition of boundaries of a taxon also exists in the biological classification of animals, but to a very much smaller degree. (There is no such thing as perfect exactness in biological concepts).

This means that we need to be humble about the present taxonomic status of ICD-10 and DSM-IV.

12.2.2 **The periodic table of elements**

Attempts to construct a classification of the chemical elements started with Antoine-Laurent de Lavoisier in 1789, when only 33 were known. The definition of an element at that time was for many years a substance that cannot be broken down further into simpler substances.

Over the next hundred years or so, as more elements were discovered and isolated in their pure forms, it became clear that they fell naturally into small groups of three or even five members, but a scheme that encompassed all of the gradually increasing number of elements did not emerge. The major change came in 1864 and the subsequent few years, when it became evident that if the greater number of elements by then known were listed in order of their atomic weight, elements with similar physical and chemical properties recurred at intervals of eight.

An English chemist, John Newlands, was the first to point out this *law of octaves,* but the idea was ridiculed at first; the then influential Chemical Society even refused to publish his work. The importance of this repeating pattern was finally recognized in 1869 and 1870 when the Russian Dimitri Mendeleev and the German Julius Meyer both published their own versions of the *periodic table.* This is particularly associated with Mendeleev, because he also pointed out that it made sense to leave gaps in the table when it seemed that there was a place for then currently unknown elements. In this way, elements such as germanium and gallium were predicted before they had been discovered.

The modern era of nuclear physics, with the realization that the atom has an internal structure, has changed the definition of an element to a substance consisting of atoms which all have the same atomic number (the atomic number is the number of protons in the nucleus), but this has resulted only in minor improvements to the same basic order of the elements in the table.

This periodic table has a very different and much simpler form from the biological classification of animals, and both its structure and the method of characterizing the elements appears to bear no relationship to anything that might be analogous in contemporary psychiatry and psychology. But there are still two valuable basic points to be noted. First, something which started off with quite crude items of information gradually changed, over a long period of time, into something powerful and sophisticated. Second, it was only when precise measurements became available, in this case measurements of the properties of atoms, that the classification of elements came to life.

To sum up, the two points that emerge from this brief consideration of both these powerful and useful classifications are quite general but nevertheless important. First, efforts to find increasingly useful ways of classifying psychiatric disorders should not be inhibited by the present necessity to use only simple descriptive data, and second, the search for reliable measurements of any type that are clearly correlated with clinical symptoms and syndromes must continue.

Notes

1   Ornulv Odegard, Professor of Psychiatry, Oslo (a man of few words but great wisdom), once said to me, 'We must not get too worried about trying to define mental disorders exactly. Many of the definitions we use are rather like the lines of latitude and longitude on a map. If you go looking for them, there is nothing there, but they are very useful for helping us to get around.' JEC.

2   Hierarchies, or sets of interdependent levels of organization, can be seen in a great many things once they are looked for. The term first came into prominence in relation to the hierarchy of angels, such as Seraphim, Cherubim, and Archangels, often mentioned in religious works. Each level in a hierarchy can be seen to have its own identity conceptually, but yet also depends upon the level below it. Similarly, each level contributes to the functions of the one above it. Hierarchies of rank and functions are essential to most human organizations, such as armies, industrial organizations, and academic units in universities. It seems reasonable to speculate that more knowledge about the hierarchies of the brain and mind will lead to a better understanding of psychological functions and psychiatric disorders. JEC.

Chapter 13

Special problems for psychiatric classification

13.1 What is being classified? Definition of disease

ICD-10 Chapter V and DSM-IV are essential as a means of communication; consequently they are used widely and regarded as successful classifications. So long as clinical psychiatrists can easily find in a classification the most common and important clinical states that they have to deal with in their daily work, they usually do not give much thought to the nature of the classification itself. Similarly, they rarely have strong views about the definition of what it is that they need to have classified. Generic terms such as 'mental illness' and 'mental disease', which delineate their field of work, have proved impossible to define satisfactorily, in spite of a long and multidisciplinary debate. These terms, and others such as 'physical illness', are useful and important in ordinary conversation, but precise definitions which indicate clear borders between, for instance, physical illness, mental illness, and social problems, have eluded psychiatrists, physicians, and sociologists in spite of debates that started in the 1950s. Barbara Wooton, a sociologist, agreed with Aubrey Lewis that social criteria should not be part of the definition of the concept of mental illness, and they both also concluded that there was no easy way of differentiating between the concepts of mental illness and physical illness (Lewis 1953; Wooton 1959). Much later Scadding, a physician, suggested that the best definition of a disease was something that produced a 'biological disadvantage', a viewpoint also favoured by Kendell (Scadding 1967; Kendell 1975). This has the disadvantage of placing homosexuality alongside such things as cancer and severe metabolic diseases, which many find unacceptable.

The trio of general concepts 'disease, illness, and sickness', without any attempt to differentiate between physical and mental aspects, has already been noted in the Introduction and Section 13.1. They are useful but overlapping concepts, particularly in many of the patients seen in general psychiatric practice, as illustrated in Figure 13.1.

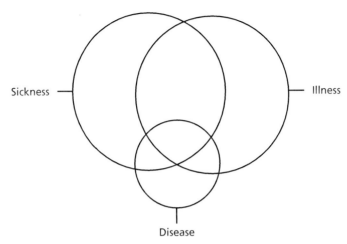

Fig. 13.1 Overlapping concepts of disease, sickness, and illness.

13.2 **What is the real job of a modern, scientifically trained doctor?**

In the background to this whole subject is the usually unstated but powerful assumption (made possible by modern medical knowledge and technology), that the real job of modern, scientifically educated doctors is only to identify and treat physical diseases that can be identified by the presence of abnormal physical signs or laboratory findings. The disease causes the patient to feel ill, which is unpleasant for the patient and family, and may interfere with activities, but these effects can be dealt with by nurses, social workers, and psychologists. If the investigating doctor has this attitude, then if all physical investigations are negative, unfortunate phrases such as 'there is no genuine illness present' can often be seen in medical notes and referral letters. Psychiatrists naturally find this attitude unacceptable, since they deal with many patients in distress and suffering from considerable interference with all activities, but who have no positive findings when laboratory investigation are carried out. This has led first Kräupl Taylor and then Fulford to suggest that *all* doctors should have a dual approach (Kräupl Taylor 1971, 1976; Fulford 1989). That is, starting with the first consultation, they should give equal priority to alleviating the distress of the patient and family, and to investigating the possible presence of physical abnormalities. Fulford has called this 'the reverse approach', but perhaps 'the parallel approach' would be more acceptable to medical educators.

The widespread consultations for ICD-11 and DSM-5 that are now under way have resulted in the renewal of the debate about the best way to define mental illness or mental disorder.

Psychiatrists are not the only ones who are frustrated by this difficulty. Lawyers, administrators, educators, and members of many other professions related to medicine and psychiatry would all welcome a brief and unambiguous definition. But perhaps the complicated and multi-dimensional nature of this group of related concepts makes a simple, one-sentence definition of any of them an impossible objective.

13.3 **The concept of a disorder**

As a way of side-stepping this problem, in both ICD-10 and DSM-IV the clinical states which constitute the work of psychiatrists and other mental health workers are called 'disorders'. Disorder is given a conveniently imprecise meaning. There is no harm in this quite practical solution, so long as users realize the nature of the problem and the reasons for it.

To arrive at a useable definition of something that has purposefully been given imprecise boundaries was an interesting task that had to be tackled by the compilers of both ICD-10 and DSM-IV. Although working separately, they fortunately arrived at definitions of 'disorder' that are broadly similar, but there is an important difference that is easily overlooked.

13.3.1 **The definition of disorder used in ICD-10**

A passage in the *Introduction to the Clinical Descriptions and Diagnostic Guidelines* acknowledges the problems noted above, and states that, 'disorder implies the existence of a clinically recognizable set of symptoms or behaviour associated in most cases with distress and interference with personal functions. Social deviance or conflict alone, without personal dysfunction, should not be included in mental disorder as defined here.'

13.3.2 **The definition of disorder used in DSM-IV**

A similar approach is adopted in the *Introduction to DSM-IV*. The same definition of disorder given in DSM-III and DSM-III-R is used, defined as follows; 'each of the mental disorders is conceptualized as a clinically significant behavioural or psychological syndrome or pattern that occurs in an individual and that is associated with present distress (e.g. a painful symptom) or disability (i.e. impairment in one or more important areas of functioning), or with a significantly increased risk of suffering death, pain, disability, or an important loss of freedom. In addition, this syndrome or pattern must not be merely an explicable and culturally sanctioned response to a particular event, for example, the death of a loved one. Whatever its original cause, it must be currently considered a manifestation of a behavioural, psychological, or biological dysfunction in the individual. Neither deviant behaviour (e.g. political, religious, or sexual) nor conflicts that are primarily between the individual and society are mental disorders unless the deviance or conflict is a symptom of a dysfunction in the individual, as described above.'

In both ICD-10 and DSM-IV it is emphasized that social deviance or conflict alone, without personal dysfunction, should not be included as a mental disorder, but there is an important difference between them. In the additional discussions about the meaning of disorder, there is greater emphasis in ICD-10 about the need to avoid, as much as possible, including interference with social functions. This is because of the marked differences in the importance of such interference in the many different cultures in which the ICD-10 will be used. The difference between impairments, disabilities, and social handicaps as defined in the ICD system becomes important for this (see Chapter 15). In ICD-10 it is also noted that a disorder causes distress or interference with personal functions 'in *most* cases'. This statement implies that there may be *some* cases in which a disorder may be recorded as present, when there is no distress or interference with personal functions. This is different from DSM-IV, where the presence of 'clinically significant distress or impairment in social, occupational, or other important areas of functioning' is regarded as a part of all disorders, and is even included as a major requirement for a disorder (for instance, criterion C for Major Depressive Episode, and criterion B for schizophrenia).

Although at times these differences may seem like trivial hair-splitting, there is a strong logical point in the background; it is surely best to avoid including the consequences of a disorder among its defining features. Unfortunately, it is necessary to include the qualifying statement 'as far as possible' because at present, the unsatisfactory nature of some concepts in ICD-10 (for instance, simple schizophrenia F20.6, mild hypomania F30.0, and some of the personality disorders) means that a few disorders can be manifest only by interference with social functioning.

13.3.3 The definition of disorder used in DSM-5

Due to the lengthy discussions about the exact wording of the definition of disorder to be used in DSM-5, this is not available at the time of writing. However, by the time this book is published, the DSM-5 will have been published, and it is likely that the definition of disorder will be broadly similar to that used in DSM-IV-TM (see Addendum, page 119).

Chapter 14

Diagnosis in psychiatry

14.1 What is a diagnosis?

This simple question is rarely the subject of choice in psychiatric teaching seminars, but is well worth raising, because to do so leads immediately into a discussion of several important issues.

Every society possesses healers who are consulted by people who feel unwell and who do not know how to get themselves better. The healer's task is to discover the cause of the unpleasant experience, by seeing through the presenting symptoms and signs, and to diagnose another different kind of process that is causing them (dia- = one apart from another; gnosis = recognition, knowledge). The healer then uses expert knowledge and skills to remove the underlying cause, and this alleviates the troublesome signs and symptoms.

Diagnoses are made in whatever terms seem useful to the healer, derived from the healer's ideas of causation of illness and appropriate treatment, based upon the same ideas. Doctors and healers of previous generations made diagnoses and gave treatment according to the medical beliefs of the time (the ideas of causation now seem strange, and some of the treatments were dangerous). Doctors of the future will make diagnoses and give treatments that we cannot at the moment even imagine.

Modern medical knowledge and technology have developed to a remarkable degree in only a few generations, so that physicians and surgeons are now often able to identify the anatomical or physiological abnormalities that underlie many types of presenting symptoms. This means that an aetiological diagnosis that indicates the best treatment has become possible for many patients. But psychiatrists are not in such a powerful position with a large proportion of their patients, because of the current lack of knowledge about the mechanisms that underlie common psychiatric symptoms such as depression, obsessions, delusions, and hallucinations. For these, a descriptive statement to indicate the symptoms or syndrome present is all that can be done, and this is called a disorder. Much more is known about the aetiology of traumatic brain damage, dementia, drug-related, and alcoholic disorders, and modern genetics is revealing what lies behind the many types of genetically caused mental retardation (learning difficulties) that are now being identified. But patients with these disorders are still only a minority of the overall psychiatric workload arising in a community.

14.2 **Components of the diagnostic process in psychiatry**

The diagnostic process in psychiatry is more complicated than most medical trainees realize. A full account of this can be found in publications elsewhere (Cooper 1983; Kendell 1983), but it is worth repeating here some basic points and a brief summary of the several stages of the process.

The diagnostic process that goes on in the mind of a clinician interviewing a patient so as to arrive at a diagnosis can be divided into a sequence of several inter-dependent stages, the most important aspects of which are:

1. The interviewing technique of the interviewer.

2. The perception by the interviewer of the patient's speech and behaviour. Some of this is spontaneous and some is in response to the interviewer.

3. A complicated series of processes in the interviewer's mind during which the information perceived is sorted out into categories which allow the interviewer to decide what to ask next, and to begin to work out how best to summarize what is wrong with the patient.

4. A final stage of classification, in which the interviewer chooses one or more terms from a psychiatric classification. This will allow the diagnosis of the patient to be recorded and communicated to others in a way they will understand.

All of these processes can be rapid and more or less automatic, and they also depend upon what the interviewer has learned from previous experience.

The small number of studies of diagnostic decision-making in clinical psychiatry have highlighted two surprising features. First, the rapidity with which confident diagnostic decisions are made, and second, a lack of awareness on the part of the interviewer as to which items of information are the important ones. Gauron and Dickinson (1966) noted that the psychiatrists they studied often formed quite definite diagnostic impressions within the first minute of an interview. Similar findings were obtained by Sandifer, Hordern, et al. (1970) and Kendell (1973). These studies were done many years ago, and need repeating and extending because they illuminate what are still quite basic clinical issues. For research purposes, however, procedures such as SCAN and CIDI have been developed which, as far as possible, make the interviewing and diagnostic processes overt, and reduce the between-observer variations in judgements. In the training courses for both SCAN and CIDI, the trainee is taught to concentrate on rating only symptoms and complaints that are clearly present, and not to jump to conclusions or make interpretations about which symptoms might or should be present because a particular diagnosis seems likely. In other words, the whole diagnostic process is made descriptive, and slowed down so that its reliability can be increased.

14.3 Making more than one diagnosis

To describe fully the clinical state of some psychiatric patients requires the use of more than one diagnosis, and it is also often found that there is some doubt about which diagnosis in a classification is the best fit for the symptoms. In these instances, the clinician should consider recording a list of possible diagnoses; this list is usually called a *differential diagnosis*. This may then need sorting out into main, subsidiary, and alternative diagnoses. The main diagnosis is the one in which there is most confidence (and usually the most obvious and the most troublesome, requiring action such as treatment or admission). A subsidiary diagnosis is not in competition with the main diagnosis; it is present but of a different nature (the commonest examples being a personality disorder or an anxiety state). Alternative diagnoses are added if there is not much confidence in the main diagnosis.

14.4 Narrative descriptions versus lists of criteria

ICD-10 and DSM-IV are classifications of categories, and for most ordinary purposes the diagnostician has to decide whether a disorder is present or absent. How this decision is arrived at is up to the diagnostician. Two contrasting approaches to making this decision are currently being widely discussed, with the preparation of ICD-11 and DSM-5 in mind. (It is important to note that this debate is about the presentation of the information about the disorders, and not about the disorders themselves or the content of the classification as a whole.) The first approach is to follow the convention in psychiatric textbooks, by the providing a narrative account of the disorders that gives prominence to the main features, and also mentions other features which may or may not be regarded as diagnostic. The second approach is to provide a list of diagnostic criteria, with instructions about how many and what combinations are required to give a diagnosis. These diagnostic criteria are limited to descriptions of symptoms and behaviour, and no interpretations are included. Such lists of symptoms are often referred to, rather optimistically, as 'operational criteria', as originally suggested by Stengel in 1960.[1]

In the current debate about this issue, the traditional narrative account approach has been given the name of the 'prototypic matching'. A very useful and easily accessible account of this debate has been provided recently by the World Psychiatric Association, with papers by advocates of both viewpoints (Maj 2011; Westen 2012).

How a psychiatric classification is presented should be determined by the requirements of the users, and if there are several types of users, then several different presentations of the same basic classification will be appropriate. The multiple version approach that was adopted by the WHO for ICD-10 was based upon this principle, in that three versions of ICD-10 Chapter V were provided. First, the *Clinical Descriptions and Diagnostic Guidelines* version (CDDG) is the main version prepared with psychiatrists in mind; in this, each disorder is described in narrative terms (WHO 1992b). The *Diagnostic Criteria for Research* (DCR-10), published separately, provides the same classification in the form of lists of criteria (WHO 1993). Finally, a shortened and generally simpler and more practical version (ICD-10-PC) was provided for use in primary care (WHO 1996).

There are probably several reasons why this multiple version strategy has not been properly recognized over the years, but it is likely that a lack of publicity is one of the most important. In the instructions and introductions to each version, the existence of these other different versions is mentioned, but it is clear that the administration of the WHO did not ensure that they were advertised and promulgated widely enough and with sufficient energy to ensure that potential users knew of their existence.[2]

There seems to be general agreement that researchers prefer lists of diagnostic criteria, and this is recognized by several of the authors of the papers noted above. In contrast, a recent 'global' survey by the WPA and the WHO found that two-thirds of the participants (practising clinical psychiatrists) regarded a diagnostic system based upon clinical descriptions as more clinically useful than one based upon lists of criteria (Reed, Correia, Esparza, Saxena, and Maj 2011). Commenting on this, Maj noted that 'the proportion of DSM-IV users endorsing this position was even slightly higher than that of ICD-10 users'.

14.5 The drawbacks of lists of criteria in clinical practice

14.5.1 The risk of an appearance of spurious diagnostic precision

Whatever the hopes and recommendations of the compilers of such lists, and however carefully they provide instructions for their use, there is no way that the users can be forced to do what they are told. This applies to experienced clinicians just as much as to trainees (Zimmerman and Gallione 2010). Anecdotally, when this problem is discussed informally with trainees, many will admit that whether they have checked each item on a symptom list or not, they still record the diagnosis as if they had, when they have a strong impression that the diagnosis is likely (particularly if they are short of time, as they often are).

Administrators, lawyers, other medical specialists, and other professionals naturally assume the best about diagnoses based upon the use of a list of criteria, and often make comments such as 'at last psychiatrists seem to know what they are doing'.

14.5.2 Reluctance to arrive at a diagnosis and start treatment

When some of the criteria listed for a diagnosis are not satisfied, and a definite diagnosis cannot therefore be made, there may be a reluctance to commence treatment even though it is obvious that the patient is very likely to benefit.

14.5.3 Reduction of the incentive to read widely

Trainees may be tempted to assume that the symptoms listed in the criteria are all that it is necessary to know about the condition. This may reduce the trainee's incentive to read widely, and to learn about important aspects of conditions that are not mentioned in the criteria. In the instructions for use provided for both DSM-IV and ICD-10, there are clear statements that these classifications should not be regarded as substitutes for textbooks and wider reading, but pressure of work, inaccessibility of libraries, and shortage of funds often lead to these warnings being ignored.

14.6 The dimensional approach

In contrast to deciding whether a disorder is present or not, an alternative way is first to describe a number of dimensions which contribute to the disorder, and then state the position of the subject on each dimension. This method depends upon knowing how to measure several independent dimensions which contribute to the disorder in question, so it is more elaborate than a simple categorical statement. In essence, these two approaches are not as different as they seem at first sight, because the definition and measurement of a dimension can only be done by first making a number of initial categorical decisions about the boundaries of the dimensions, and the definition of the intervals on the scales by which the dimensions are to be measured. At the present time, this approach is really a non-starter, because for most psychiatric disorders there are still no independent dimensions that can be measured. As knowledge progresses, there will probably be a requirement for both approaches in an overall classification, but for the moment the simpler categorical style is the most practical, particularly when clinical decisions about case management have to be made quickly, sometimes on the basis of incomplete information. On the whole, researchers are likely to try to develop dimensions that can be measured, whereas clinicians will probably continue to prefer the ease and speed of decisions that come with categories.

14.7 **Participation in the development of classifications**

There is often a problem in getting the voices of clinicians heard during the development of classifications for general use, even though clinicians are the main users of such classifications. The great majority of committees or task forces on the development of classifications are composed of keen researchers, often specialists in a limited field of disorders, who are naturally motivated to ensure that the group of disorders about which they know the most are fully accommodated. This means that they usually have little interest in how things fit together to form the classification as a whole.

Another problem is that the most vocal critics of a classification often have comparatively little knowledge of, or interest in, the principles of classification that need to be followed as far as possible by all sections of the classification. The most common example of this is that primary care physicians often complain that the classification they are asked to use is not based upon either aetiology or the need for particular treatments, which are their main concerns in daily clinical work. This is why the diagnostic features of each category in the primary care version of ICD-10 are accompanied by notes on several topics, including possible medication. However, this extra information is presented in a way that makes it clear that it is there for the convenience of the user, and that treatment and management are not (and cannot be) part of the classification itself (WHO 1996).

14.8 **Lumpers and splitters**

A debate between 'lumpers' and 'splitters' is almost always part of the development of a classification of anything, and has been particularly prominent in the biological sciences. Lumpers try to create coherent groups, and are prepared to ignore small differences to achieve this. Splitters emphasize differences, and seek smaller and highly differentiated groups that have no exceptions. Whether you are a lumper or a splitter depends partly upon the subject matter being classified, and partly upon your personality characteristics.

Progress towards better psychiatric classifications needs an optimistic and tolerant approach to both of these tendencies; splitters might be able to identify new methods and mechanisms that can help to form the basis of new groups of disorders, and lumpers may be able to define new ways of grouping disorders together that lead to new concepts. But suggestions must be accompanied by or suggest new ways of measurement associated with the new ideas put forward.

Recent examples of lumping are at present being widely discussed as preparations are made for ICD-11 and DSM-5 (Andrews, Goldberg, Kreuger, et al. 2009) (see chapter note 1 in Chapter 19). Up to now, these new groups are not based upon any new measurements or fresh concepts, so it is difficult to see how they might lead to improvement in the classifications. Nevertheless, exploration of this type of suggestion should be encouraged, and it would certainly be a good idea if the same major headings could be used for both DSM-5 and ICD-11.

Notes

1 Strictly speaking, the word 'operational' implies that a measurement has been made, in addition to a reliable description being provided. Nevertheless, to describe a symptom or item of behaviour in a way whose reliability can be tested is as good a substitute for measurement as can be achieved at the moment.

2 In the background of this problem is the fact that the remit of the WHO is to produce a variety of health-related documents for use by its member states, but it is not obliged to do any more than inform the official office of government publications of each member state of the existence of such documents. The WHO headquarters and its technical divisions produce formal documents in the six main languages of the WHO, and other documents (e.g. guidelines and technical documents) in English. Some of the technical documents are also produced in other languages, but not all. Publications that reach a government office are therefore not necessarily reaching the professional community that should be the main user of some of the documents and materials that WHO produces. That this is so was well demonstrated by the publication of the ICD-10 classification of mental disorders translated into German and published by a commercial company—the sales of the classification were very significant.

Chapter 15

Classification beyond the diagnosis

15.1 Limitations of the diagnosis

> When physicians dismiss illness because ascertainable disease is
> absent, they fail to meet their socially assigned responsibilities.
>
> *(Eisenberg 1977)*

This brief comment (by an American social psychiatrist) leads the way into a
discussion of a number of issues which illustrate how the fears and hopes of
patients who feel ill are often left unsatisfied by a statement from the doctor
that they do not understand (such as a unexplained diagnostic term). Even
worse is a statement that a diagnosis cannot be made because investigations
have shown nothing positive. Unless the doctor accompanies this type of
statement by reassurance that the patient's symptoms and illness will still
be taken seriously, this can easily be interpreted by the patient as meaning
that the doctor will now lose interest in providing some sort of help. Patients
and families are usually worried by the possibility of a prolonged period of
unpleasant symptoms, or of disability and dependence, and the technical
terms of the investigations or of the diagnosis may have little meaning to
them. (There are, however, some circumstances in which the pronounce-
ment of an impressively worded diagnosis can be welcomed by the patient
and family, even though they have no idea what the terms mean. This can
happen when, after seeing several doctors who all tell them that they can
find nothing definitely wrong, the patient is seen by yet another doctor who
gives a diagnosis using words of which they have never heard. This may be
a great relief because it gives the impression that they have at last found a
doctor who knows what he is talking about.)

Because it is comparatively easy to collect diagnoses of patients from
the medical case-notes, diagnostic classifications are often used for purposes for which they are not suitable. The most common example of this
is when administrators require a measure of costs of an episode of illness.
Unfortunately, the costs of treatment and care for an episode of illness are

not as closely correlated with diagnosis as is often assumed. This is because the length and severity of the illnesses of different patients with the same diagnosis may vary widely. As populations age, and new and ever more expensive treatments are developed, administrators need more realistic methods of costing health services and care systems than just a diagnosis can provide.

Clinicians must ensure that administrators and non-clinical managers understand that a diagnosis is only one part of the overall description of the patient's illness. The 'Diagnosis-Related Groups' (DRGs) of the Medicare and Medicaid systems in the USA and other estimates of costs of care based only upon diagnosis are a poor substitute for properly designed and applied measures of actual care consumed. An additional problem is that unless busy clinical staff are given special training, and part of their time is set aside for the purpose, the information they are able to collect will not be accurate or complete enough to form the basis of valid statements about costs and degree of disability. This point seems to be very relevant to the 'clustering' rating system recently introduced in the UK as part of the 'payment by results' approach to the recent restructuring of the National Health Service (Royal College of Psychiatrists 2012).

15.2 The illness, the person, and interaction with other persons

One of the deficiencies of the psychiatric classifications currently in use is that almost all of their constituent disorders are described as being manifest by symptoms and behaviour of just one person. Exceptions to this are some of the personality disorders and the disorders of childhood and adolescence, but there are a number of other disorders in which disturbances of relationships with other persons are almost always prominent and well recognized in practice, without this being recognized in the classifications. For instance, some of the somatoform disorders could just as well be seen in a wider context as disturbances of illness behaviour and the sick role (Cooper 1999). This has been recognized by some authors in publications with titles such as *Illness as a Way of Life* (Ford 1983), and 'Allergic to Life' (Simon et al. 1990). There are now signs that DSM-5 (and perhaps ICD-11) will contain a much more prominent recognition of this wider context. In *A Research Agenda for DSM-V*, the chapter on personality disorders contains some 20 pages of discussion about 'relational disorders' (Kupfer, First, and Regier 2002). It is to be hoped that something positive on this will appear in DSM-5 in due course.

15.3 **Disability**

A full discussion of the description and classification of disability is beyond the scope of this book, but some brief comments are justified. Severity and length of periods of disability are some of the most obvious contributors towards the burden of illness upon the patient and family, and the overall costs of care. This whole topic also suffers from the problem that up to now, it has been customary in the medical and related professions to regard terms such as impairment, disability, and handicap as interchangeable. But accurate use of any system of description requires more careful and consistent use of these terms than is needed in everyday medical or social conversations.

This has been recognized by the development of descriptive classifications that divide disability into several sub-types, such as impairment of mental and physical functions, difficulties in performing everyday 'activities of living', and social handicaps. The most highly developed of these is the International Classification of Functioning, Disability, and Health (ICF), published by the World Health Organization. This is presented in both long and short forms (WHO 2001a and b).

The ICF has a hierarchical structure, and much care has been taken to ensure that categories are clearly defined and do not overlap. (An outline of the ICF is given in Appendix 3.) It covers a wide range of interpersonal and social interactions, and takes into account the ways in which the activities of an individual are influenced by the immediate environment. In many ways it is a considerable improvement on its predecessor, the International Classification of Impairments, Disabilities, and Handicaps (ICIDH) (WHO 1980). Nevertheless, even the short version requires careful study before it can be understood and used correctly. This is not the fault of the schedule, but is simply due to the fact that the satisfactory description of disability is a large and complicated subject, involving a wide range of possible human activities and interactions with environments.

In the USA, a system of rating disability in the context of rehabilitation, devised by Nagi, has also been popular among neurologists (Nagi 1965), but it seems likely that the ICF will now be used increasingly.

Chapter 16

Multi-axial classification

16.1 First attempts

The complete assessment of a psychiatric patient and family requires enquiry into more than just the diagnosis; other aspects such as previous personality, level of intellectual ability, social situation, relationship problems, and the presence of disability may be crucial to formulating a management plan. The idea that these should be systematically recorded at the same time as the diagnosis has been around in the psychiatric literature for many years, but has come into prominence only comparatively recently. Perhaps this recent interest is in part due to the development of modern information technology, which allows an increase in the amount of information that can be recorded at little or no extra cost. Another likely influence is the wish to educate psychiatrists and others using the classifications about the importance of contextual factors, disability, and the general health conditions of patients being assessed.

The first publications about multi-axial classifications appeared many years ago; in 1919 Kretschmer recommended that for each case, in addition to the diagnosis there should be a note about the causal factors, such as the characterogical, organic, and psychosocial factors influences (Kretschmer 1919). Some 30 years later, Essen-Möller and Wohlfahrt produced a proposal for a system that would allow the coding of the diagnosis and the causal factors (Essen-Möller and Wohlfahrt 1947). A few years later Bilikiewicz proposed a triaxial system that would allow the recording of the diagnosis, the causal factors, and personality characteristics (Bilikiewicz 1951). Leme Lopes in 1954 went even further, suggesting that there should be an axis that would deal with treatment and another to record the legal implications (Leme Lopes 1954). Ottoson and Perris then took Essen-Möller's proposal and added axes that were to serve for the recording of the course of illness and the severity of the condition. (Ottoson and Perris 1973). Helmchen then proposed a pentaxial classification which was to include certainty of the psychiatrist about the diagnosis (Helmchen 1980). Mezzich also produced a very useful review of this whole subject (Mezzich 1979).

These, and some other proposals for multi-axial classifications (including the proposal for a tri-axial classification of mental disorders in children made in the framework of the WHO programme on standardization of psychiatric diagnosis), contained interesting and useful ideas, but apparently had no general effects.

There is no sign in the literature that multi-axial classifications are in general use by psychiatrists. This is probably partly because there are so many competing ideas and partly because the use of the multi-axial classification requires additional work without a direct incentive or return.

16.2 **DSM-III and ICD-10**

The situation changed in 1980 when the American Psychiatric Association decided to introduce a multi-axial system in DSM-III, the third revision of its diagnostic and statistical manual. DSM-III was presented as a multi-axial classification, and so were DSM-III-R, DSM-IV, and DSM-IV-TR. The axes for DSM-III were:

Axis I Clinical psychiatric syndromes (and V codes from the ICD system, entitled 'Other conditions which may be the focus of clinical attention').

Axis II Personality disorders and development disorders (including mental retardation).

Axis III Physical disorders and conditions.

Axis IV Severity of psychosocial stressors.

Axis V Global assessment of functioning *(special scale provided)*.

The same axes have been used for all versions of the DSM.

Similarly, two multi-axial schemes have been produced for use with ICD-10. These are:

1. The WHO Multi-Axial Classification of Child and Adolescent Psychiatric Disorders (WHO 1966). This has six axes:

   (a) Clinical psychiatric syndrome

   (b) Specific disorders of psychological development

   (c) Intellectual level

   (d) Co-existent medical conditions

   (e) Associated abnormal psychosocial situations

   (f) Global assessment of disability

2. The WHO Multi-Axial Classification of Adult Mental Disorders (Janca et al. 1996; WHO 1997). This has several innovative features. It abandons the division between mental and physical disorders, placing any and all disorders on the first axis. This confirms the WHO's official

position that mental and physical disorders should be considered as of equal importance, and so given equal attention. The second axis deals with circumstances that may influence the illness and its presentation. The innovation here is that the axis uses the Z code chapter of the ICD, instead of having a specially devised list. The third axis records the overall level of disability, regardless of the cause or causes, and uses the already existing WHO schedule, WHO DAS 2. After tests of reliability and ease of use carried out in more than 30 countries, the classification was published.

Two other multi-axial schemes were planned by the WHO but did not reach completion. One was to record mental health problems in the elderly, and the other to record problems encountered in primary care. Both of these encountered problems during their development, although a preliminary report on the primary care scheme was published (WHO 1992).

The Cuban Psychiatric Association proposed a multi-axial classification (using six axes—clinical disorder, disability, adverse environmental factors, personality, maladaptive mechanisms and tests, and therapeutic responses), but it is not certain what proportion of psychiatrists in Cuba use it. The Chinese Psychiatric Association also produced a multi-axial classification in the 3rd Revision of the Chinese Classification of Mental Disorders (CCMD 3, Chen 2000). The seven axes of that classification include, in addition to axes that correspond to the axes of the DSM, two more axes. One deals with global clinical impressions and one with inter-relation among the ratings on the other six axes.

16.3 Are multi-axial classifications used widely in clinical practice?

Multi-axial classifications seem to be so sensible that one might expect to find some publications from several countries describing their use, and perhaps even assessing whether they have the beneficial effects upon the standards of case-note keeping and patient care that might be expected. There is, however, a dearth of such studies, and the few that there are suggest that multi-axial classifications are used infrequently. Two surveys (Banzato and Rodrigues 2007; Mellsop et al. 2007) showed that less than one-third of the psychiatrists who used the DSM-IV system used all the axes. The use of the ICD tri-axial system has been reported by an even lower percentage of psychiatrists who declared that they are using the ICD classification.

Informal enquiry leads to the same conclusion, and suggests that even in teaching hospitals and units, the psychiatric trainees are rarely required by their seniors to make full use of a multi-axial system for the routine recording of the clinical state of their patients. It is possible only to speculate why this might be so, but among the likely influences are: (a) there is no positive financial incentive to do so; (b) there is no penalty for not doing so; (c) for trainees there is usually a considerable pressure of work which makes the simple recording of the diagnosis an easier option; (d) in a modern multi-disciplinary team, the information that would go into the non-diagnostic axes is often collected by non-medical members of the team; although many aspects of the patient and family are discussed in meetings, nobody has the responsibility of ensuring that this is all recorded in the case-notes.

The multi-axial system for child and adolescent psychiatry seemed to suffer the same fate, even though it was put together and recommended by the leading child psychiatrists of the day. It is also possible that research workers find that although the topics they are investigating are mentioned in the axes, they are not dealt with in sufficient detail for special studies; the research teams therefore construct their own schedules and scales. Nevertheless, it is probable that the prominence given to multi-axial schemes by prestigious bodies such as the APA and the WHO, has had a generally good effect on clinical work. It has reminded clinicians and trainees of the importance of considering many aspects of their patients and families in addition to the traditional medical emphasis on the diagnosis.

In 1988 at the start of the long programme of development of ICD-10, J.D. Burke noted that there was some doubt as to whether many clinicians in the USA were actually using DSM-III when arriving at the diagnosis of their patients (Burke 1988); he quoted from a study dated 1984 that diagnosis by DSM-III was 'often praised but seldom practised' (Jampala et al. 1986; Skodol 1987). Perhaps the same will be said of multi-axial classification.

It is difficult to foresee what is likely to happen to multi-axial classification in the future. For the moment, it can be said that multi-axial classification seems to be a very good idea that has probably had a good general influence upon clinical practice, but has not yet fulfilled its early promise.

Chapter 17

Psychiatric classification in a wider perspective

17.1 National and international classifications

Stengel's 1960 report for the WHO, published in 1960, illustrated the chaotic situation of the immediate post-war period, as already noted in Chapter 1. The years that followed saw a gradual recognition worldwide of the need for international agreement on a classification that would serve as a 'common language', and the WHO programme provided this in the form of ICD-8 Chapter V and its glossary. Since then, ICD-9 and ICD-10 have been widely accepted and used, although a few countries have made a few minor modifications for local use. A recent survey carried out by the Zonal Representatives of the World Psychiatric Association confirmed that most of the previously existing national classifications are no longer in use and those that are, such as the 3rd Revision of the Chinese Classification of Mental Disorders, are very close in both structure and content to the ICD classification. A notable exception to this is the DSM system, a series of classifications produced by the American Psychiatric Association. In addition to their use within the USA, these have become popular internationally, particularly for the publication of research papers in internationally recognized journals.

17.2 Properties of an international classification

At the start of the preparations for ICD-10, the following requirements for an international classification were listed (Sartorius1988):

1. It must be based upon points of agreement between mental health professionals.

2. It must be sufficiently simple and understandable to allow its easy use by those who will deal with commonly encountered disorders.

3. It must be sufficiently well-liked as a tool of information exchange to be easily translatable into any already established national classifications.

4. It must be rather conservative and theoretically familiar so as to be attractive or at least acceptable to a wide variety of users of different levels of knowledge and backgrounds.

5. It must be stable, and subject to change only when sufficient scientific knowledge has become available to openly justify any innovations.

6. It must take into account languages into or from which it will be translated.

7. Between successive revisions, there must be considerable continuity, for both economic and scientific reasons.

The criteria by which psychiatric classifications might be assessed are also discussed in detail in an excellent review by Jablensky and Kendell (2002).

One of the main purposes of the ICD is to facilitate the publication of health care statistics by all member countries that can be used to describe the state and, as time passes, the development of health services. As one of the 21 chapters of the whole ICD, Chapter V must also conform to the basic ICD rules that allow comparison between regions and countries (the names and numbers of the chapters of the whole of ICD-10 are given in Appendix 4). All chapters must have a defined size and structure; for ICD-10 this is an alpha-numeric decimal structure (each chapter has both a letter and a number). Chapter V(F) of ICD-10 was allotted ten two-character categories, and three major three-character categories; each of these can be subdivided if required into ten four-character categories. There are no particular psychiatric or scientific reasons why disorders should be divided into ten groups or a hundred sub-groups, but in practice these rules do not cause any serious problems because of the large amount of classificatory space now available.

The nomenclature of the ICD will always be likely to contain terms considered by doctors of some countries to be of doubtful value, simply because they are considered to be important in other countries with well-established traditions. When each revision of the ICD is considered to be complete, the final version then has to be approved by the political bodies that govern the WHO; these are the Executive Board, a Revision Conference, and the World Health Assembly. The latter brings together the Ministers of Health of all the WHO member countries.

The ICD also has to be suitable for translation and use in many languages, which is not the case for national classifications. The DSM system has always been an exception to this, and the APA promotes the translation of its classifications into a number of languages; this has been particularly so for DSM-IV. It is likely that similar efforts will be made to ensure that DSM-5 will be widely known and used. Fortunately the efforts to bring the ICD and the DSM classifications together which began with the development of ICD-10 and DSM-IV have continued, so that the latest versions of the two classifications now in preparation should be even more similar.

17.3 **Meta-effects of classifications**

Clinical psychiatrists tend to think of a psychiatric classification as something they have to use when recording the diagnoses of their patients. A classification is also something that they were taught as trainees, and one of the things that they teach their juniors. It is also something that they refer to if involved in research. But in addition, an officially recognized classification also has important effects upon:

1. the work and education of all other mental health professionals

2. the recording and work of health administrators and managers

3. sickness benefit systems

4. mental health legislation and the work of the legal profession

5. the public and inter-professional image of psychiatry and psychiatrists

6. the stigma attached to most psychiatric diagnoses and activities.

These and other related issues are discussed in detail in Appendix 4, which is a chapter entitled 'The Meta Effects of Classifications' by N. Sartorius, in *The Conceptual Evolution of DSM-5* edited by D. Regier (2011). It is reproduced here by kind permission of the American Psychiatric Association.

Chapter 18

How to use a psychiatric classification

18.1 The future uses of the diagnosis and case-notes

What is the point of recording a diagnosis and case-history in the patient's notes and hospital records? The best approach to answering this question is to remember that information entered in the hospital or clinic records is not only for the psychiatrist and others caring for the patient. It is also for the benefit of the patient and carers in the future, so that if the patient has a relapse or recurrence of the illness, it will contribute towards the best possible decisions about treatment and management.

18.2 How to use a psychiatric classification badly

What does a psychiatrist do when using a classification badly?

(This section is placed first because it is probably close to what many psychiatrists do when they have to record a diagnosis in the case-notes or hospital records for patients they have seen in their daily clinical work.)

1. The psychiatrist thinks about the patient, and if the memories about the patient are rather hazy, has a quick look through the case-notes.

2. The psychiatrist thinks about the classification, and tries to remember which of the categories fits the patient best. If the knowledge of the classification is also hazy or incomplete, the psychiatrist then chooses a category that, as far as can be remembered, more or less fits the patient, and records it as the diagnosis.

3. If a little more time is available, the psychiatrist may actually look up the category which seems to fit best, but reading only the titles and the list of diagnostic criteria in the pocketbook publication of whichever classification is being used. The psychiatrist ignores the longer description of the conditions which (in both the DSM-IV and the ICD-10 full versions) precedes the lists of criteria, and may include the associated features and points about the differential diagnosis.

4. So long as some of these criteria seem to have been present, the category is recorded as the diagnosis.

18.3 **How to use a classification properly**

1. In an ideal world, the education of the psychiatrist (both general medical and postgraduate psychiatric) has included acquiring some knowledge of the general principles of classification. The psychiatrist has realized that in the present state of psychiatric ignorance about basic causes and processes of psychiatric disorders, all contemporary psychiatric classifications are imperfect, but necessary for communication about patients.

2. The psychiatrist has already learned the main categories and sub-categories of the classification to be used, and has read the various warnings and instructions for use provided by the compilers of the classification in the introductory sections.

3. The psychiatrist first reads the case-notes, noting the most prominent recent symptoms, and then reads (in the full form of the classification), the description of the most likely category that fits the patient. If sufficient symptoms are present, then the diagnosis is recorded. The confidence of the main diagnosis should be recorded, in a short narrative comment about how well the patient's clinical state fits the description given in the classification.

4. If the patient has additional prominent symptoms which make an alternative or an additional diagnosis possible, then these are also recorded, together with a brief narrative comment pointing out what has been recorded and why. (This is best done as noted in Section 14.3 under the heading 'Differential diagnosis'.)

18.4 **Learning and teaching**

Approached in this way, the making and recording of a diagnosis becomes a constructive learning experience (and if done with a trainee, a teaching experience). This is because to arrive at a diagnosis shows what features a patient has in common with other patients, and also often emphasizes ways in which the patient is unique.

18.5 **All classifications are imperfect**

Patients are rarely a perfect fit to the categories of a classification, and with clinical experience comes the realization that no existing classification is perfect. Classifications should be used as helpful guides when making clinical decisions, but should never be used rigidly. They pick out some features of individuals, but can never give more than a partial picture of any individual person. To know both the imperfections and the strengths of currently used classifications should be part of the everyday knowledge of all well-educated psychiatrists.

Chapter 19

The future

19.1 The development of ICD-11 and DSM-5

As this companion is going to print, work is still in progress on the proposals for the classifications of mental disorders to be included in the 11th Revision of the International Classification of Diseases (ICD-11) and on the finalization of the proposals for the Diagnostic and Statistical Manual, 5th Revision (DSM-5). The table of contents of DSM-5 has already been released into the public domain, and can be found at http://www.psychiatry.org/dsm5.

The full DSM-5 will be presented and on sale in May 2013 during the Annual Convention of the American Psychiatric Association in San Francisco. At that time, the ICD-11 chapter on Mental and Behavioural Disorders will still be in the process of production. It is likely to be finished in 2014 so as to be presented to the World Health Assembly for approval in 2015.

The process of developing the new revisions of the DSM-5 resembles the process used in the development of proposals for the ICD-10, as described in Section 10.3. The APA approached the production of the proposals for the DSM-5 in a similar way. It first convened several meetings to review basic issues related to the classification (Kupfer and Regier 2002) and continued—with the support of the USA's National Institutes of Mental Health, Alcohol, and Drug Abuse—with a series or scientific review meetings involving leading experts from the USA and from other countries. The latter made nearly one-third of the total attendants at these conferences. The results of these conferences served as background materials for the consideration of the APA DSM-5 Task Force (Beach, Wamboldt, et al. 2006; Sunderland, Jeste, et al. 2007; Narrow, First, et al. 2007, Dimsdale, Xin, Kleinman, et al. 2009; Andrews, Charney, et al. 2009; Regier and Narrow 2011; Saxena, Esparza, Regier, et al. 2012).

The Task Force created a number of working groups which then proceeded to work on the proposals for groups of disorders. Once the proposals were produced, field tests of the classification were conducted and their results served as background material for the production of the final proposals of the DSM-5 submitted to the governing bodies of the APA.

The World Health Organization created an advisory group that was to help the Division of Mental Health and Substance Abuse Control to produce its proposals. The advisory group created working groups which will prepare the proposals to be considered by the advisory group and then finalized. In collaboration with the World Psychiatric Association, the World Health Organization has also carried out a survey of opinions asking psychiatrists in different parts of the world about their experience with the ICD-10 and about their views concerning the ICD-11 (Reed, Mendonça Correia, et al. 2011). In addition to the working groups that examined the different groups of disorders, the WHO has also established a working group that is to produce proposals for the classification of mental disorders to be used in primary health care. It is hoped that the proposals of this latter group, working in parallel to the other groups, will be in harmony with the classification that will be included as a chapter in the ICD-11. In order to harmonize the proposals for the DSM-5 and ICD-11, officials of the WHO and APA have met on a number of occasions. They agreed on a 'meta-structure of the classification' which will be used as a guide in the finalization of the proposals for the two classifications (Andrews, Goldberg, Kreuger, et al. 2009).[1]

19.2 **Conjectures on the future of classifications of mental disorders**

The future of the classification of mental disorders would not present so many problems, nor would it need so many revisions, if scientific investigations were to produce evidence that would allow the formulation of the 'true' classification of mental disorders. The situation would then be similar to that concerning the classification of elements which are all accommodated in the periodic table of elements. This is unlikely to happen. Neither psychopathology nor genetics are anywhere near that level of knowledge, and medicine—and in particular psychiatry—will have to keep producing classifications of disorders summarizing the knowledge available at the time of their making. These successive versions of the classification will continue to be no more than hypotheses about the true relationships between disorders and we shall have to discard them whenever new knowledge makes this possible and necessary.

There are, however, changes in the context of the classification of mental disorders which will make the task of creating new and useful classifications more difficult than was the case with the classifications produced until now. The first of these changes relates to the technology of information processing. Immensely powerful, the new information systems allow the recording of considerably more data about people with mental disorders who are receiving care and it is not impossible to imagine that in the future diagnoses will be replaced by diagnostic formulations as units of classification.

Similarly the technology would allow the recording of dimensional profiles of mental disorders and of summaries of information until now rated on the axes of the classification, the linkage of information about the current episode of illness with previous episodes, and the presentation of the state of the mentally ill person in new graphic methods. Whether psychiatrists and other users of the classification will be willing to 'feed' the information systems is an open question that can only be answered once it is clear what incentives will be used to make them do so.

A second major change of the context in which the classification is to be used is the divergence of the areas of interest of specialists and those less specialized. The fragmentation of the psychiatric profession is clearly a trend that will continue in the future—in part because of the vast increase of knowledge which cannot be easily handled by a single person and in part because of academic and political reasons—such as the promotion in one's career and notoriety in the professional and lay circles which goes with virtuosity in a particular area. Thus, in addition to specialists in mental disorders of children and in the elderly, there are now specialists in mental disorders in women, in diseases of migrants and refugees, and in the ailments of adolescents. In addition we already see psychiatrists who are specialized in bipolar disorders, in schizophrenia, in anxiety; even those groups are now split into those who are specialized in the early forms of illness and those interested in its long-term course. The hope that the division between biologically oriented and psychologically oriented psychiatrists will diminish has not been realized; in addition to the previous division there are now further subdivisions by preferred method of treatment or some other criterion. There is a danger that the classifications that these subgroups of specialists are going to develop and use will not be understood nor used by anyone but themselves. The notion that these super-specialist classifications have to be translatable into a main classification which will allow the communication among all the subgroups as well as between them and the specialists in other parts of medicine may not be popular, and there may be a lamentable lack of effort to maintain the linkage with a central classification.

On the other end of the spectrum—in the organization of care at primary care level—the recognition that a great deal of psychiatric practice occurs in general practice has led to the development of classifications for use in primary health care; while in the beginning these were linked to the 'mother' classification the more recent forms of classifications for primary care have already moved away in their development and form from the main classification so that they cannot be translated into it. This is true both for the classification produced by the general practitioners (e.g. the WONCA-produced ICPIC—the International Classification of Mental Disorders for

Primary Health Care) and for those produced by psychiatrists for use by general practitioners.

A third challenge to the universal use of a classification of mental disorders stems from the current steady decline of interest in the discipline of psychopathology. The number of psychiatrists who are choosing psychopathology as their main area of work is diminishing and their ardour to understand and describe symptoms and syndromes as well as their relationships seems to be vanishing. This is a paradoxical trend in view of the variety of new forms of symptoms of mental disorders. Migrants from rural to urban areas and those from different countries show new forms of symptoms reflecting the mixing of the cultural backgrounds of the donor and the recipient communities: although specialists in cross-cultural psychiatry have described some of these symptoms, thorough psychopathological descriptions and analyses of these symptoms and clinical conditions are still lacking. Syndromes linked to the new technological world—such as various forms of internet addictions—are also awaiting an in-depth psychopathological analysis which until now is not forthcoming.

New knowledge will also have an influence on the future of the classifications of mental disorders. As was the case with some disorders which were previously in the chapter of mental disorders and then changed their place once new knowledge about them became available (e.g. the 'general paresis of the insane') it can be expected that certain mental disorders until now solidly in the field of psychiatry will 'migrate' to other areas of classification, e.g. because their pathogenesis brings them closer to other groups of disorders than to psychiatric problems. Depressive disorders, for example, might be the consequence of inflammatory processes which under the influence of a variety of factors might lead to diabetes: if it turns out that diabetes and depression indeed share a common pathogenetic process, their placement in a classification of diseases will have to be re-examined and this might lead to significant changes of the classification.

It is to be hoped that these and other factors will not lead to the disappearance of a single, central classification of mental disorders into which all other classifications made for specific purposes can be translated. The acceptance and use of a single 'mother' classification is a prerogative for communication and collaboration in the field of psychiatry and in the field of medicine. Sir Aubrey Lewis in the 1950s spoke of a public health classification that should be common and used by all, and of specialists' classifications responding to needs of different professions, research, and services: perhaps he should have also added that any special classifications should also be translatable into the public health classification without losing too much information.

Notes

1 The meta-structure proposed divides the disorders in the classifications into five clusters:

1. Neurocognitive disorders (identified principally by neural substrate abnormalities).
2. Neurodevelopmental disorders (identified principally by early and continuing cognitive deficits).
3. The psychoses (identified principally by clinical features and biomarkers for information processing defects).
4. Emotional disorders (identified principally by the temperamental antecedents of negative emotionality).
5. Externalizing disorders (identified principally by the temperamental antecedent of disinhibition).

This 'metastructure' has had some influence on the major headings used for DSM-5, and is also likely to be reflected in ICD-11.

Appendix 1

Foreword to *The Glossary of Mental Disorders and Guide to their Classification*

Compiling glossaries has been a respectable profession since the 2nd century BC, as the article in the *Encyclopaedia Britannica* makes abundantly clear. This is not surprising when the multifarious needs for classification and interpretation are considered. But there is a reverse side to the coin: to 'gloss over' or 'to gloze', a term derived from the same root as glossary, denotes a disreputable activity. 'Classification' likewise has a pejorative as well as a respectable flavour. Psychiatric usage of the relevant terms attests their ambiguity: 'mere labelling', 'the neat complacency of classification', 'nosological stamp collecting', 'a medical hortus siccus'. Such damning phrases arise, in part, from revulsion against the excesses to which classification was pushed in the late 18th and early 19th centuries.

A modern psychiatric glossarist has to cope basically with the same uncertainties and pitfalls as beset the compilers of other medical classifications, but they are aggravated by hazards arising from the paucity of the objective data on which definition and diagnosis must depend. He has to contrive appropriate criteria for differentiating one disease from another; ideally he aims at constructing a consistent schema into which they will all fit. Such a schema may be based on clinical patterns (syndromes) or on clinical course; it may be psychodynamic, etiological (genetic), or pathological. And, since diseases are in any case abstract concepts, it is no wonder that the disease constructs with which psychiatrists work have shimmering outlines and overlap. Observer variation is disconcertingly in evidence; reliability is too low for scientific comfort; discrepancies may be in some cases lessened, in others minimized, depending on whether they arise from inexact perception, personal bias, or divergency of the nosological systems or terms used.

The picture is no longer black. The glossary put forward here, when faithfully applied, reduces the scope of error. It would seem, however, that accurate observation is still the gate that needs the closest guard. A. R. Feinstein put it bluntly: 'the current psychiatric debates about systems of classification, the many hypothetical and unconfirmed schemas of "psychodynamic mechanisms", and the concern with etiological inference rather than observational evidence are nosologic activities sometimes reminiscent of those conducted by the mediaeval taxonomists'. Since the disorders listed in this glossary are identified by criteria that are predominantly descriptive, its use should encourage an emphasis on careful observation.

This glossary still contains some compromises and anomalies, but the emergence of an agreed version from an international group of collaborators and advisors of such diversity of background and outlook was possible only because of a generous spirit of cooperation and common recognition of an urgent need for better means of communication.

Sir Aubrey J. Lewis, M.D., F.R.C.P.

Foreword to the *Glossary of Mental Disorders and Guide to their Classification,* for use with the *International Classification of Diseases,* 8th revision (1974). By Sir Aubrey J. Lewis. M.D., F.R.C.P. Reproduced with permission from the World Health Organization.

Appendix 2

Some results from the US/UK Diagnostic Project

The US/UK Diagnostic Project teams studied a series of 250 consecutive admissions to Netherne Hospital in London and Brooklyn Mental Hospital in New York. The findings were subsequently confirmed in sample surveys covering all the state and area mental hospitals in the two metropolitan areas. The project psychiatrists worked in the hospitals under the same conditions as the hospital psychiatrists, but without communicating with them in any way. The mental states of all patients were assessed by means of the then recently developed Present State Examination, 8th edition (PSE-8). The 'project diagnosis' was a consensus diagnosis using the British Glossary to the 8th edition of the International Classification of Diseases of the World Health Organization (ICD-8). Spitzer's DIAGNO computer program was used as check on the consistency of the project diagnoses (Spitzer and Endicott 1968; Cooper 1970). These procedures allowed the project diagnoses to be used as a standard against which the diagnoses of the British and American hospital psychiatrists could be examined. This was not meant to suggest that the project diagnoses were correct or absolute, but simply meant that they were made according to stated procedures and criteria and were as free as possible from variations between the diagnostic concepts of the psychiatrists.

At Brooklyn, the project team made far fewer diagnoses of schizophrenia than did the hospital staff (29.7% for the project against 56.6% for the hospital), but many more diagnoses of affective illness (36.6% for the project against 16.6% for the hospital). At Netherne, the project team again diagnosed schizophrenia less often than the hospital staff, but to a lesser degree (22.8% for the project team against 35.2% for the hospital staff). At Netherne, the project team also made more diagnoses of affective illness than the hospital staff (58.6% for the project team against 46.2% for the hospital staff). In summary, the staff of both the American and British hospitals diagnosed schizophrenia more readily than did the project staff, but this tendency was much more marked at Brooklyn. For affective disorders, the staff of both hospitals made the diagnosis less readily than did the project staff, but again this tendency was more marked at Brooklyn.

The London–New York comparison

The findings of the Brooklyn–Netherne study were so striking, that it was considered necessary to carry out a second and wider Anglo-American comparison to find out if the results could be generalized with confidence. In this second study, a sample of 192 patients admitted to the nine mental hospitals serving New York, and a sample of 174 patients admitted to 18 of the mental hospitals serving Greater London were studied, using the same project staff and procedures. This study is described in detail in the Maudsley Monograph No. 20 (Cooper, Kendell, Gurland, Sharpe, Copeland, and Simon, 1972).

The findings were substantially the same as those of the Brooklyn–Netherne comparison.

Appendix 3

The WHO International Classification of Functions, Disability, and Health (ICF)

The ICF is the successor to the International Classification of Impairments, Disabilities, and Handicaps (ICIDH). This was presented as a classification of the consequences of diseases (WHO 1980), and it was mainly concerned with the consequences of physical diseases. This means that the sections covering mental disorders were not well developed. Nevertheless, it was used in many countries. At first glance, the ICF looks similar to the ICIDH, but it is actually more comprehensive and its coverage of the consequences of mental disorders is much better than the ICIDH. Its unit of classification is 'categories within health and health-related domains'. This means that the ICF does not classify people, but describes the situation of each person within an array of health or health-related domains, and always within the context of environmental and personal factors. It is intended to be a classification of 'components of health', and takes a neutral stand with regard to aetiology. It is published in a short form and a full form; anyone considering using the ICF is recommended to start with the short form, before deciding whether to move on to use the more detailed full form. Study of a paper giving the background of some of the concepts involved would also probably be helpful (Bickenbach et al. 1999).

The ICF has two parts, each with two components:

Part 1 Functioning and disability

    (a)   Body functions and structures

    (b)   Activities and participation

Part 2 Contextual factors

    (c)   Environmental factors

    (d)   Personal factors

Each component can be expressed in both positive and negative terms.

Each component consists of various domains and, within each domain, categories, which are the unit of classification. Health and health-related states of an individual may be recorded by selecting the appropriate category code or codes, and then adding *qualifiers*, which are numeric codes that specify the extent or the magnitude of the functioning or disability in that category, or the extent to which an environmental factor is a facilitator or barrier.

The short form of the ICF is accompanied by considerable detail and guidance about how to use it. A great deal of effort was put into ensuring that the many lists and details of the components are complete. At the very least, the ICF can be used by any of the caring professions as a source of useful check lists, to ensure that all the important aspects of persons (either with or without medical problems) and their interactions with environments have been considered.

The meta effects of classifying mental disorders

This is a chapter by N. Sartorius, in *The Conceptual Evolution of DSM-5* edited by D. Regier, W.E. Narrow, E. A. Kuhl, and D.J. Kupfer (2011).

During a meeting convened by J. Zubin in 1959, C.G. Hempel presented his paper on classification, and in the discussion that followed, A. Lewis suggested that it is necessary to distinguish two types of classifications of mental disorders (Fulford and Sartorius 2009). One type is *public* classifications: these should serve to improve communication between all concerned and might be the best to use in epidemiological and other research, where researchers want to make their findings comprehensible and comparable with findings of other scientists. The other type is *private* classifications, which serve the needs of particular groups that have reached agreement on the use of names for categories and their content. Public classifications should 'eschew categories based on theoretical concepts' and be 'operational and descriptive'. It would then be possible to communicate and compare results of epidemiological studies.

A public classification of mental disorders has to satisfy scientific, public health, and practical requirements. Scientific requirements include a need to make the classification reflect scientific evidence; a need to satisfy taxonomic requirements (e.g. that the categories of the classification should be mutually exclusive and jointly exhaustive; i.e. they should allow the placement of each of the objects of the classification into a single category, and the total of categories should make it possible to place all objects that are being classified); and an effort to preserve continuity between the revisions of the classification so as to permit comparisons over time (Sartorius 1976). Practical and public health requirements include a need to make the classification easy to use in practice; a need to ensure that the public classification has links with 'private' classifications (and that it can be translated into different languages and into classifications used by other professions, e.g. psychiatric nurses); and a need to reflect experience, particularly if evidence is not available. Until now, in the classification of mental disorders, the practical requirements have been easier to satisfy than the scientific: the knowledge about the pathogenesis of mental disorders is still insufficient to govern the structure of the classification, and satisfying some of the taxonomic requirements would have made the classification less easy to use and therefore unlikely to be generally used. The purpose of the International Classification of Diseases (ICD), from its original version to its most recent revision, ICD-10 (WHO 1992b), has been to facilitate communication of, and comparisons among, findings. The ICD should be seen as a typical example of a public classification that classifies data in a manner that makes it possible for all those interested—governments, researchers, and practitioners—to understand and compare facts relevant to healthcare. In the beginning, the ICD was no more than a list of categories that grouped causes of death. Gradually the remit for the ICD was expanded to include diseases, reasons for contacting services, disability, health care interventions, and other facts of importance for planners and practitioners of health services (Sartorius 1995).

A classification of diseases, including the ICD, is produced to facilitate reporting about activities of health care services and epidemiological estimates of parameters of diseases (e.g. their frequencies) in populations. Classifications and their productions, however, also have other uses and effects. Classifications contribute to definitions of the medical disciplines, including psychiatry. They can be used as a basis for health insurance and related public health measures.

They also can have significant effects on the images of medical disciplines and on the perceptions of people with diseases included in these classifications. Classifications, which are used as bases for training health personnel, usually become platforms for action and learning in later life. Finally, classifications also can define directions of research, sometimes restraining innovative scientific explorations of issues that cut across the categories of the classifications. In this chapter, I examine these remote effects of classifications of mental disorders. However, before doing so, I briefly discuss four problems that face the makers of classifications of mental disorders.

Problems facing makers of classifications of mental disorders: What should be grouped?

The English language has the luxury of a choice of four terms for psychiatric maladies. These words are used loosely, but it is accepted generally that the word *illness* refers to the experience of a person who has the malady, the word *disease* to a medical substrate of the malady, and the word *sickness* to social recognition of the malady, for example, in determining sickness benefits (Sartorius 2002).

The problem that plagues psychiatry—or at least is better recognized in psychiatry than in other medical disciplines—is that the areas covered by these three terms overlap only in part (see Figure 13.1).

Some people feel *ill*, although it is not possible to detect a medical substrate, a tissue damage, that would justify the use of the word *disease*, whereas some people with *diseases* who have major tissue damage or other medical findings do not feel *ill*. Some people are declared *sick* and given treatment even though they have no signs of *disease* and do not feel *ill*, a sad phenomenon that finds its acme in the abuse of psychiatry for political purposes. It is not always clear what should be grouped in a classification: ICD-10 has labelled the conditions seen in psychiatric practice *disorders*, a vague term that denotes the incomplete overlap of the three meanings of malady just described (WHO 1992b).

Caseness and diagnoses

A second problem that psychiatry (and its classifications) has to face is that there is a difference between a psychiatric diagnosis and 'caseness'. Whether someone is a 'case' depends on the purpose of this label. Thus, in epidemiological studies, a case might be defined differently from a case in assessment of psychiatric services or in estimation of the need for service or intervention. The difference between a case and a psychiatric diagnosis lies in the use of the three dimensions of 'caseness': (1) the cluster of symptoms that psychiatry considers as the disease; (2) the distress that an individual who has the disease experiences; and (3) the disability—the impairment of functioning—that the disease produces, in the context of an individual's life situation, personality traits, and, possibly, co-morbid diseases. Here again, overlap between the syndrome, the distress, and functional impairment can be significant, partial, or non-existent. Some people with a particular form of a disease are disabled by it, whereas others are not. Some people are severely distressed but do not show the symptoms necessary to satisfy the definition of a disease. A person who discovers a wart of black colour might be severely distressed because he or she fears that the wart is an early stage of a melanoma that will spread rapidly, although he or she is neither disabled nor has a disease. Other persons might be disabled to a severe level but show few symptoms of a disease. The cluster of symptoms, the disability, and the distress can each be measured in terms of severity, and it is probable that extreme severity of any one of the three dimensions of caseness will make those persons (or their caregivers) seek help from health services or others who surround them even if they have no (symptomatic) diagnosis.

In some classifications of mental disorders—notably, the Diagnostic and Statistical Manual of Mental Disorders (DSM)—the definition of a mental disorder requires the presence of symptoms, disability, and distress. This is a problematic solution because of a growing amount of evidence that the impairment of functioning of people with mental disorders depends much more on social class, personal assets, cultural expectations, and other factors than on disease alone. The ICD recommends to users of the chapter on mental disorders that they should not use disability (*functional impairment* in the language of DSM) in making a diagnosis of mental disorders because disability depends, to a large extent, on the social environment of the person who has the disease. ICD, however, also uses impairment in the performance of basic functions (e.g. self-care) as a component criterion for some conditions (e.g. the dementias). Clinicians often attempt to help persons who seek help because they are severely distressed but are not disabled or showing sufficient symptoms to be diagnosed as having a mental disorder. The question that will have to be resolved soon, in order to inform the compilers of ICD-11 and DSM-5, is whether the classifications should group diagnostic terms or 'cases' seen in psychiatric and general medical practice.

Consequences of ignorance about the pathogenesis of mental disorders

Another major problem for makers of the classifications is that of the relationships between disorders that are to be grouped. Two, or more than two, morbid events can be considered as parts of the same disorder if their pathogenesis is the same. Thus, if the pathogenesis of depression is the same as the pathogenesis of anxiety, the two conditions should be considered the same, not co-morbid, despite the fact that their clinical pictures are different. For example, in ICD-10, retinopathy, peripheral neuropathy, polydypsia, and keto-acidosis are all grouped in categories assigned to diabetes because they share a common pathogenesis. The term *co-morbidity* should be reserved for instances in which two morbid events of different pathogenesis exist in the same individual at the same time.

The pathogenesis of most mental disorders is still a matter of speculation and remains largely unknown. Consequently, at present, the classification has different categories for conditions that might be the same in their pathogenesis and, vice versa, the classification wrongly groups disorders of different pathogenesis into the same category. The same situation applies to uncertainty about the way to deal with the reappearance of morbid events that have similar symptoms in the same person: if the pathogenesis of the morbid events results in the same clinical picture on each occasion, the classification should place them into the same category, counting them, for epidemiological and treatment purposes, as one disorder. If the pathogenesis is different on each occasion (although the clinical condition and symptoms may be the same), the events should not be counted as episodes of the same disorders but as independent diseases, somewhat like injuries that can occur for different reasons many times in the course of one's life.

For the time being, it has been decided to classify psychiatric disorders by their symptoms; this decision is not necessarily the best, but it seems to be the only one possible in the current state of our ignorance. This classification choice has the advantage that the grouping of disorders can be done reliably: among its disadvantages is that such a classification can be reified, taken to reflect the natural order of things, although it is no more than a hypothesis of the real nature of mental disorders created on the basis of evidence available at a point in time (Sartorius 1988). When this happens, the classification can, in fact, hamper the exploration of pathogenetic processes involved in the syndromes that modern operational criteria have placed together into categories.

Overlap between variants of lifestyle, impairment, and mental disorders

Variants of lifestyle and behaviour that are seen in people with mental disorders may overlap. Persons, such as the famous 'clochards' of Paris, who have chosen to live on the street without permanent abode and rely on charity, often do not have demonstrable mental disorders; yet vagabondage has been included as a category in the classification of mental disorders in some countries. Also, in recent years we have seen the exclusion of homosexuality from the classification of mental disorders in ICD-10 and in some national classifications, whereas in other classifications homosexuality still is seen as a mental disorder that requires psychiatric treatment. Hermaphrodites have raised their voices, protesting that their condition is described as a disorder of sexual development (Karkazis and Feder 2008). People with intellectual disability are opposing the notion that their conditions should be classified in the chapter on mental disorders in the ICD under the name of mental retardation. In some countries, hazardous driving has come to be seen as an expression of a mental disorder that should be removed by psychotherapy. These examples of conditions that have been placed into the classification of mental disorders or removed from it illustrate a difficulty that is specific for the makers of such classifications.

Areas of mental health programs affected by the classification of mental disorders and their revisions

The identity of psychiatry

A medical discipline is defined by the disorders that it treats, by the methods that it uses to treat such disorders, and by the length of time necessary to learn how to use these treatment methods. Therefore, any discussion of a classification of mental disorders also is a discussion of the identity of psychiatry. The classification indicates whether a particular disorder 'belongs' to psychiatry, and the totality of the disorders placed in a classification of mental disorder defines the limits of psychiatry. If all disorders that are currently classified in the classification of mental disorders were to be moved to other chapters of a classification of diseases, psychiatry would cease to exist.

This relationship between the classification of mental disorders and the identity of psychiatry—and thus also of psychiatrists—makes it certain that a discussion about classification will be of great interest to psychiatrists, raise emotions, and lead to intense discussions and anxieties. Clinicians who represent other medical disciplines are, of course, also interested in the matter, because the definition of the territory of one discipline usually affects the territories of others.

The controversy surrounding the concept of sub-threshold disorders exemplifies the way in which classification of mental disorders influences the definition of the discipline of psychiatry The existence of sub-threshold disorders is a by-product of the use of operational criteria that define categories of mental disorders on the basis of a consensus rather than evidence. The term sub-threshold disorders came into existence when the classification of mental disorders was 'operationalized'—that is, when the American Psychiatric Association published DSM-III (APA 1980a), in which each category of the classification was provided with a description of criteria that had to be satisfied, if a disorder was to be placed in that category.

It places before psychiatrists a dilemma that will be difficult to resolve. As things stand, it is clear that psychiatrists who provide treatment to people who do not have a disease (but have a sub-threshold disorder) could be seen as fraudulent charlatans because they treat people who do not have disorders. However, if these psychiatrists do not help people who come to them with sub-threshold disorders—for example, people who do not show many symptoms but are very distressed—the psychiatrists are not fulfilling their roles of good physicians. Also, problems related to sub-threshold disorders are close to problems related to states that show some similarity to mental disorders but are considered different from them and therefore should not receive psychiatric treatment, such as grief reactions, excessive religious zeal, and related behaviours (e.g. self-flagellation and even crucifixion).

Psychiatrists, as well as other physicians, often see patients who ask for help because of problems that might be causing distress or impaired functioning. Psychiatrists examine these patients, advise them, and provide treatment that is not necessarily different from treatment that would be provided to a patient who has an 'above the threshold' disorder. These clinicians are helping people who are distressed or disabled but who do not have all the symptoms that have been selected to define a category. In other medical disciplines, the threshold of illness usually can be expressed in terms of laboratory findings or results of a variety of examinations that provide 'hard data', such as those obtained by the use of X-ray or imaging apparatus. Psychiatry does not have that luxury, and helping people who do not meet criteria (set by psychiatrists!) of illness can easily lead to the accusation that psychiatry medicalizes the problems of daily living so that its practitioners can make money.

Another example of the effect of changes of classification on the definition of the discipline of psychiatry is the removal of the 'progressive paresis of the insane' from the classification of mental disorders (now placed with the communicable disease chapter, because it is a late form of syphilis). It is true that other medical disciplines deal with conditions for which diagnosis is based mainly on patients' complaints (e.g. migraine and some other forms of headache), but the numbers of such conditions in other chapters of the classification of diseases is much smaller than for psychiatry.

By removing the condition from the chapter 'belonging' to psychiatry, the discipline has, in fact, unofficially been declared unable to deal with behavioral syndromes caused by a communicable disease.

The second descriptor of a discipline—a definition of methods that its practitioners will use—also depends on the definition of disorders and their grouping in the classification. If disorders that are grouped in a category (because presumably they have the same pathogenesis) do not react in the same way to the methods of treatment that define psychiatry, it is legitimate to doubt the effectiveness of such methods and, by implication, the justification for the existence of the discipline that uses them. Johannes Reil, who introduced the term *psychiaterie* some 200 years ago, argued that the discipline of psychiatry should be created in order to demonstrate that mental disorders are not moral failings or consequences of black magic but diseases like any others and that it is therefore necessary to create a medical discipline that will demonstrate that both diseases of the body and diseases of the mind are the legitimate subject of medicine (Marneros 2004). Methods used in the treatment of physical illnesses have similar effectiveness for all the disorders grouped in a category of the classification. If this does not hold for psychiatry, it becomes difficult to see psychiatry as a discipline similar to its sisters in the practice of medicine. The vagueness of the limits of psychiatric disorders, and of the categories in which they are placed, as well as a reluctance to define precisely what methods of treatment psychiatrists should or should not use, has allowed the emergence of territorial disputes with practitioners of non-medical disciplines and others—for example, practitioners of alternative medicine. These disputes are considerably more important in the field of psychiatry than in other parts of medicine. Such disputes are often settled politically, with decision-makers disregarding the option of assessing which professional group is best qualified to provide care and deciding, on the basis of that evidence, who should be doing what.

Financial resources for health care of persons with mental disorders

The recent decision to introduce parity in the reimbursement of health care expenses for mental and physical disorders in the United States was considered, justly, an important step to more equitable treatment of people with mental illness. People with conditions placed outside the DSM-IV (APA 1994) chapter on psychiatry have not had any disadvantage in terms of reimbursement, even if their conditions were disorders that, in other classifications, would fall into the chapter that groups mental disorders (e.g. premenstrual dysphoric disorder and postviral fatigue syndromes). On the other hand, in some countries—for example, in Eastern Europe and Vietnam—psychotic mental disorders have been treated free of charge, whereas patients have had to pay for treatment of other mental, and most physical, disorders. Psychiatrists have often indicated that patients had psychosis so as to ensure that treatment was free even though the psychiatrists knew the patients had other conditions.

These examples indicate the influence of a classification on the funding of health care on an individual level. On the level of societies' decisions about health care, a classification also plays an important role. During the preparation of ICD-10, there was a long and intensive discussion about the placement of cerebrovascular disorders. Neurologists argued that the consequences of stroke made it highly probable that such patients would come under their care; cardiologists argued that the conditions were due to vascular damage, and therefore the disorders should be placed in the chapter on cardiovascular disorders. However, the background of the argument was not exclusively scientific. Finally, stroke was placed into the chapter on cardiovascular diseases, and its consequences, such as hemiparesis, were placed into the chapter on neurology. As a result, in calculating mortality, stroke is reported as a cardiovascular illness.

Many governments make decisions about the distribution of resources on the basis of mortality figures. Diseases that kill more people are given higher priorities in national health programs and thus receive more resources. Cerebrovascular disorders are a major cause of mortality; thus, their placement in the classification underlines the importance of the discipline that deals with people with the condition that causes death.

In some instances, when it was too difficult to decide where to place a condition, a special arrangement was introduced into ICD-10: the same condition was placed in two chapters. One placement carried a sign of a dagger, indicating that death due to that disease should be coded in that chapter, whereas the other placement carried an asterisk, indicating that care provided to a person with the disease should be coded in that chapter. Thus, for example, dementia found its place as a cause of death in the chapter on neurological disorders and as a cause of treatment in the chapter on psychiatric disorders.

The definition of categories affects estimation of prevalence of disorders, another dimension that decision-makers take into account when assessing the priority and financing of healthcare. A broad definition of a category will increase the total number of cases that can be considered as being in need of care; narrowing a category (i.e. making criteria more stringent) will decrease prevalence and incidence estimations for conditions placed in that category and will have a negative influence on the priority given to the discipline responsible for the care of people with such diseases.

HIV/AIDS provides another example of the role that a classification might have on resource allocation. Although HIV is a neurotropic virus and persons with AIDS often experience depression and, later in the course of the illness, dementia, both HIV-related dementia and encephalopathy are included in the chapter on infectious diseases; depressive states observed in the course of the illness are not specifically identified. Resources given to the fight with HIV/AIDS have been vast, but it is not easy to direct a reasonable amount of these resources to research on psychiatric and neurological components of the syndrome or to the provision of care for people with psychiatric and neurological problems linked to their HIV/AIDS. Researchers in Africa will often include a reference to HIV/AIDS in proposals for mental health research and service support, because this will make the acquisition of funds considerably easier; they will get funds that they would not get if they wrote their proposals without mention of AIDS.

These examples illustrate the effect of a classification on reimbursement and on decisions about priority of health programs. In the eyes of the decision-makers, psychiatry deals with disorders that are not very frequent, are long-lasting, and usually do not respond to treatment. Psychiatric disorders are not seen as contributing to mortality: suicide and violent acts linked to mental disorders are not placed in the chapter dealing with mental disorders but in a different chapter. Therefore, mortality due to these causes usually does not enter into the decision-making as an argument for higher priority of mental health programs.

The image of psychiatry

For a long time, a majority of the population (including a sizeable part of health care workers and political decision-makers) considered most mental illnesses to be incurable. Persons who had a mental illness were seen as being of little value for society, and because they were not curable, it seemed logical that society should be reluctant to invest money in the provision of adequate care or to support a medical discipline that seemed incapable of diminishing the prevalences of mental diseases or improving their courses. The main reasons for providing any support, therefore, have been the obligation of a society to help its feeble members and the need to protect society from the evil deeds of the mentally ill. The ethical imperative—helping members of society who are feeble or in distress—often has lost out in competition with other causes of social action.

The second reason for action—protection of society—was satisfied by measures such as incarceration or involuntary hospitalization of mentally ill people, often under conditions that would speed up their demise. Psychiatrists were seen as ineffective in the treatment of mental illness and as serving primarily as guardians of patients in the institutions. With the advent of psychoanalysis, psychiatrists came to be seen as a luxury the rich could use to unburden their worries. Not infrequently, psychiatrists have been seen as having diseases similar to those seen in their patients: this opinion has been another part of the rather poor image of psychiatry.

The classification of mental disorders also plays a role in stigmatization of the discipline of psychiatry. This begins with a medical education and the puzzlement of medical students who do not understand why they have to learn about 670 disorders (currently the number of categories used for the classification of mental disorders, according to ICD-10) when there are so few types of medications (i.e. antidepressants, anti-psychotics, tranquillizers, and stimulants) used for treatment of all these disorders. In the eyes of a medical student, psychiatrists who have produced such a classification cannot be practice-oriented doctors, an impression that is further strengthened when students hear about matters such as the necessary duration of psychoanalytic psychotherapy and the abuse of psychiatry for political purposes. The vagueness of language used by some psychiatrists in describing the categories of their classification of mental disorders (and principles used to make the classification) is, for these students, further confirmation of the fact that psychiatrists are neither real doctors nor particularly useful consultants. Once students complete their medical training, graduates usually maintain their opinions about various disciplines of medicine, including psychiatry, and contribute to the dismal image that psychiatry has for the general public. The removal of categories of mental disorders from the classification of mental disorders as soon as the cause of the mental disorder is found (e.g. the AIDS dementia and general paresis in the chapter on communicable diseases) further strengthens doubt that psychiatry is a medical discipline. If it were a real medical discipline, the argument goes, then conditions that are presenting psychiatric symptoms, but are the result of a 'real' (physical) illness, should be treated by psychiatrists, like other disorders for which there is no certainty about a physical cause as yet. Doubt about whether psychiatry is a part of medicine also is enhanced by the reluctance of psychiatrists to deal with physical illness. The existence of specialists of 'consultation psychiatry' or 'liaison psychiatry' is a sad confirmation of this attitude. There is no specialty of 'consultation orthopaedics' or 'liaison ophthalmology': an orthopaedic surgeon is supposed to know enough about orthopaedic problems that might emerge in the practice of other doctors and the same is true for the ophthalmologist who is expected to be able to deal with issues concerning his or her discipline regardless of the ward on which the patient is located. Among psychiatrists, on the other hand, only a precious few—the liaison psychiatrists—seem to be able and willing to deal with mental illness in people who also have a somatic illness. The media and the general public like classifications that are simple and tell them what kind of interventions are likely to be useful. Burns are divided by severity into four groups, defined by their risk to life and likelihood of reparation. Cancer, as well as cancer pain, has been classified in clear groups that are staged, and the stages have been linked to specific treatments. Communicable diseases are divided according to the bug that causes them. A number of bone and joint diseases have been precisely defined in a manner that facilitates treatment. Psychiatry, for a long time, did not produce clear and simple instructions about placement of diagnoses into categories of a classification of mental disorders. Several psychiatric disorders have been operationally defined in the past, but until the appearance of DSM-III there was no widely accepted classification that clearly stated criteria used to place a disorder into a category. DSM-III was a major step forward in improving the image of psychiatry. The next step, providing a clear specification of methods to be used for treatment of disorders that are clearly defined, has yet to be taken. It will not be easy to do this; although detailed guidelines for the treatment of mental disorders are numerous, these guidelines do not all say the same thing. Many of the guidelines express the views of their authors regardless of what other authors have said (or found); this is a situation similar to that which was described by Stengel in the 1960s, when he found that 'any psychiatrist worth his salt produces a classification of mental disorders' (Stengel 1960). Half a century after Sir Aubrey Lewis's suggestion that a public classification should have clearly defined categories, there is almost universal agreement on the need to have a classification with operational definitions of mental disorders usable in everyday clinical practice, and there is a fair amount of agreement on criteria that should be used. It is to be hoped that agreement on treatment of these conditions will not take another 50 years.

Research into the pathogenesis of mental disorders

A classification of mental disorders should be a reflection of the current state of knowledge about relationships among events, conditions, or objects that are classified. As long as it is seen as a summary of past knowledge that guides all future exploration (rather than as a rigid framework), a classification is useful; once it gets reified and is seen as the governing frame, it will stifle investigation and reduce chances of discovery of relationships between conditions or their causal links and pathogenesis.

Unfortunately, this is already happening. Enthused by the precision of definition for categories of mental disorders produced in the latter part of the 20th century, many people took the fact that diagnoses could be made more reliably as proof of their validity and of the validity of the classification that contained categories for the placement of such diagnoses. Editors of scientific journals no longer accepted papers that described research carried out on well-defined conditions unless the definitions used coincided with definitions in DSM-IV and DSM-IV-TR (APA 2000). Authorities who approved the use of medications and other treatments requested proof that a new drug was useful in the treatment of a particular condition defined in DSM-IV. One could imagine a drug with a positive effect on a certain proportion of people (who perhaps share a genetic basis) with different clinical syndromes that are classified in different categories of DSM-IV: it would be difficult to carry out research on such 'cross-category' effectiveness and even more difficult to get a licence to market a drug that helps some patients in different categories of the classification. For pharmaceutical companies engaged in the search for new drugs, it has become foolish to carry out research on a dimension of illness present in several disorders that currently are placed in different categories of DSM or ICD, because it would be impossible to obtain a licence for a drug not linked to the treatment of a condition with a particular diagnosis. In view of the fact that much of the research on psychopharmacology today is financed by the pharmaceutical industry, the classification that is now officially recognized does impede innovative research. The restrictive effect of the classification—clearly seen in the scarcity of publications that describe research on mental disorders across categories or of research on a particular dimension of mental functioning in physical and mental illness—will not necessarily be removed by a dimensional approach to the classification of mental disorders; but if that approach were to be accepted, it would, for a while, open new avenues of research (and possibly allow a different, less-stigmatizing organization of services for the mentally ill). Insofar as research is concerned, clearly it will be necessary to continue work on standardization of assessment of various aspects of mental disorders (e.g. symptoms, dimensions, or even more elementary descriptors of mental states), avoiding the obsessional adherence to diagnosis or criteria for categories of a classification. Such an approach will facilitate the discovery of pathogenetic mechanisms and thus more likely lead to classifications in which distinctions between mental illnesses are made on a scientific basis.

Stigmatization of people with mental illness

The classification of mental disorders plays an important role in attribution of stigma to a diagnosis and the individuals who have such a disorder. Mental disorders are stigmatized and generally seen as conditions that diminish the value of the affected individual for society. The image of a person with a mental illness is that of someone with symptoms, such as delusions and hallucinations, who is usually dangerous and unable to con-tribute to society; placement of a diagnosis in the chapter on mental dis-orders will make those with such a diagnosis share the negative image that frightens the public and results in many disadvantages. Recent research on stigmatization of the mentally ill has produced evidence that stigmatiza-tion of mental illness is present in a large majority of all societies and that the consequences of stigmatization are negative in all of these societies (Sartorius and Schulze 2005). Therefore, it is not surprising that people with mental illness usually hide their diagnoses and that they try—whenever they become organized—to take their diagnoses from the chapter on mental dis-orders into some other chapter of the classification. Pressure groups (often composed of patients and their families) in some instances have succeeded in avoiding stigmatization by insisting on their diagnosis being placed in a category in a chapter 'belonging' to another discipline. Thus, in ICD-10, the diagnosis 'fatigue syndrome' is in the chapter on mental disorders, whereas the less-stigmatizing term 'post-viral fatigue syndrome' has been placed in the chapter on communicable diseases. Premenstrual dysphoric syndromes found their place in the chapter dealing with gynaecological problems. The aforementioned HIV-related mental disorders are in the chapter dealing with infectious diseases. Attempted suicide is in a chapter separate from that dealing with mental disorders, although suicide and attempted suicide are usually associated with mental disorder. 'Personality type A', regardless of its severity, is placed in the 'reasons for contact' chapter, far away from the personality disorders group in the chapter on mental disorders. The diag-nosis of homosexuality has vanished from the chapter on mental disorders, although it is still considered as an abnormality (regardless of whether it is ego dystonic or not) requiring psychiatric attention in a variety of countries. There is one notable exception to this rule. Post-traumatic stress disorder, characterized by psychiatric symptoms, is the only disorder that does not seem to stigmatize a person who has it. The diagnosis is taken as an honour-able badge confirming that the bearer has gone through difficult times and that he or she deserves society's support and recognition of merit. In Japan, the previously used name for schizophrenia has been changed to a term that is considerably less frightening—from 'split mind disease' to 'thought inte-gration disorder'—and the description of the disease has been significantly changed. The positive effect of this change—for example, that doctors feel that it is easier to tell a patient his or her diagnosis and discuss treatment much more effectively—should make the developers of a classification sys-tem take the connotation of terms used in psychiatry into account, both in naming categories and in producing the criteria that will define them. This has not been done in the past: the growing power of patient and family organizations might be of major assistance in the search for terms that will not only be precisely defined but also acceptable to all those concerned.

To avoid stigmatization by a label of a mental illness, and the consequences of the stigma, patient and family organizations have sometimes taken extraordinary steps. For example, in France, an organization of families of people with mental illness lobbied and finally succeeded in reclassifying mental illness from a disease to an 'invalidity.' This classification change will allow families and patients to receive more support; however, this support comes at a cost of making the image of mental illness worse, effectively telling the general public that impairment related to mental illness is there to stay and that treatment of mental illness can do little to make people who have it recover and become valuable members of their communities.

Education of health workers

Over the past several decades, psychiatrists, proud of the significant increase in their knowledge, have continued to make the classification of mental disorders more and more complex. The number of categories has increased, and fixing their boundaries has required development of a complex system of inclusion and exclusion criteria. The detailed classification is usually not directly relevant to the choice of treatment. Thus, for example, the international classification of mental disorders now has some 60 categories for classification of various forms of depressive disorders, although treatment for all categories is similar.

A public classification, in Sir Aubrey Lewis's sense, should be simple, easy to remember, suitable for use in practice (e.g. provide some guidance about treatment) and epidemiological research, and amenable to tests of reliability and clinical utility (i.e. give guidance for treatment or other care interventions). It also should have face validity in the sense that it allows the easy and reliable categorization of most diagnoses made in practice.

The World Health Organization attempted to satisfy all users by producing three versions of the ICD-10 classification: (1) a version for research (this would be closer to a 'private' classification in Sir Aubrey's sense); (2) a version for clinical work, suitable for use by specialists in psychiatry; and (3) a version for use in primary health care. The latter has 22 categories, chosen because they are frequently seen in primary health services, can be reliably diagnosed, and can be linked to specific advice about treatment. Thus, this third version also could serve as a teaching tool in the education of various categories of health workers who are not psychiatrists.

At present, unfortunately, most health workers are educated about psychiatry and the management of mental disorders on the basis of curricula with more complex classifications and by teachers oblivious of the consequences that presentation of such classifications will have for the care of mentally ill people both in the immediate future, when the health workers complete their training, and in the more remote future, when the students assume important decision-making positions in the health care system. What health workers learn in the course of their general training is rarely updated; therefore it is not surprising that decision-makers the world over have an image of psychiatry (and of the best way to develop mental health programs), that is based on their training from many decades in the past. They were taught psychiatry on the basis of a classification of mental disorders created in the late 19th and early 20th centuries. That classification was created based on observations in mental hospitals at that time, and it served the purpose of reporting about mental illness in those institutions very well. The world, and our knowledge about mental illness as well as the practice of medicine, has changed meanwhile; yet decision-makers trained decades ago think about the organization of mental health services, as well as about evaluation of these services, using theoretical constructs implied by the classification used in teaching psychiatry in schools of health personnel when they were students. The delayed effect of teaching about psychiatry is not exceptional for psychiatry or other medical disciplines. It is therefore important to produce classifications of mental disorders that will take this delayed effect of medical school instruction into account. The 'public' classification of mental disorders, with characteristics described earlier, might serve that purpose, and this remains a major challenge for the makers of international and national classifications of mental disorders.

The abuse of psychiatry

An international 'public' classification that describes the categories of mental illnesses clearly could play an important role in preventing the abuse of psychiatry, which is sometimes supported by national classifications or classifications produced by a particular school of thought. The abuse of psychiatry for political purposes in the Soviet Union, for example, was supported by the existence of a classification that was developed in the United Soviet Socialist Republics and served to organize psychiatric care and treatment. This classification had categories with diagnoses that could be given to political dissidents and that led to the forced and harmful application of medication and other 'treatment' measures. The universal acceptance of an international classification of mental disorders based on the best available knowledge could remove the legitimacy of such actions and help to make psychiatry a useful medical discipline, immune to abuse for political, financial, or other purposes. The existence of such a classification also could serve to improve the quality of care offered to people with mental illness and to prevent abuse of psychiatry for other purposes. The introduction of new categories into such a classification, or any change of the classification, would have to be subjected to a serious examination of the evidence that underlies the reason for the change. At present, the process for doing this is not specified sufficiently. It is not at all clear how much, and what kind of, evidence would be necessary and sufficient in order to accept a proposal for a change of a category, for a change of criteria defining a category, or for a change of hierarchy of categories. Thus, commercial and personal motives may lead to the acceptance of changes that are not particularly well supported by evidence and that happen too rapidly; this means that it will not be possible to ensure that a single form of the classification is universally accepted and used.

Coda

Revisions of the classification of mental disorders are necessary when new knowledge becomes available and when there are significant changes in the health system that the classification is meant to serve. A revision of the classification is usually made by paying great attention to the formal features of the classification and congruence of the revision with the best available evidence and experience. Thus, revisions of a classification produced in this sense can reflect current knowledge about a group of diseases and can satisfy the epistemological strivings of its makers. However, a revision of a classification also has a number of remote effects that usually receive far too little attention in the process of revision. For example, a classification of mental disorders:

- affects the definition of psychiatry and the profession of psychiatrists.

- influences and changes the nature of stigmatization that bears heavily on people with mental disorders and their families.

- affects funding for mental health care and education of health care workers.

- exerts a powerful effect on directions that research into the pathogenesis of mental disorders will take and on the relative importance of findings of such research.

Therefore, it is to be hoped that the process of revision of the ICD and important classifications such as DSM will include a way to consider these remote meta effects of a revision before their finalization and introduction as one of the basic elements of health services systems, research, and education related to psychiatry and to medicine in general.

Appendix 5

International Statistical Classification of Diseases and Related Health Problems 10th Revision

The following is a list of ICD-10 codes.

Table A.1 ICD-10 codes

Chapter	Blocks	Title
I	A00–B99	Certain infectious and parasitic diseases
II	C00–D48	Neoplasms
III	D50–D89	Diseases of the blood and blood-forming organs, and certain disorders involving the immune mechanism
IV	E00–E90	Endocrine, nutritional, and metabolic diseases
V	F00–F99	Mental and behavioural disorders
VI	G00–G99	Diseases of the nervous system
VII	H00–H59	Diseases of the eye and adnexa
VIII	H60–H95	Diseases of the ear and mastoid process
IX	I00–I99	Diseases of the circulatory system
X	J00–J99	Diseases of the respiratory system
XI	K00–K93	Diseases of the digestive system
XII	L00–L99	Diseases of the skin and subcutaneous tissue
XIII	M00–M99	Diseases of the musculoskeletal system and connective tissue
XIV	N00–N99	Diseases of the genitourinary system
XV	O00–O99	Pregnancy, childbirth, and the puerperium
XVI	P00–P96	Certain conditions originating in the perinatal period

(*Continued*)

Table A.1 (Continued)

Chapter	Blocks	Title
XVII	Q00–Q99	Congenital malformations, deformations, and chromosomal abnormalities
XVIII	R00–R99	Symptoms, signs, and abnormal clinical and laboratory findings, not elsewhere classified
XIX	S00–T98	Injury, poisoning, and certain other consequences of external causes
XX	V01–Y98	External causes of morbidity and mortality
XXI	Z00–Z99	Factors influencing health status and contact with health services
XXII	U00–U99	Codes for special purposes

International Statistical Classification of Diseases and Related Health Problems 10th Revision. (http://apps.who.int/classifications/icd10/browse/2010/en). Reproduced with permission from the World Health Organization.

Appendix 6

Glossary of terms (with annotations about other closely related terms)

The meanings and explanations given here are recommended for use in the context of mental health activities. However, they are not necessarily universally accepted. In addition, the same terms may have slightly different or wider meanings in other contexts.

Complaints. These are what the subject says in reply to questions about how they feel or what is bothering them most. These initial complaints may be different from what a psychiatrist might record as symptoms, after asking further questions about intensity, frequency, and timing, and other circumstances.

Cross-questioning. The questioner takes a positively active role, asking an unlimited number of questions. This can be done in a polite and sympathetic manner, as in a clinical interview about events or the presence of symptoms. When done in a more aggressive manner, it begins to resemble what sometimes happens in a court of law or police investigation.

Definition. A statement or set of statements that indicate what a thing is, and also how it differs from other things that at first sight may seem very similar. To be useful, a definition should list and describe those characteristics of a thing that give it its uniqueness. In psychiatry and psychology, there is often a problem in trying to keep such statements short and few in number. However, in spite of the virtues of brevity, it may be wise to accompany definitions by extra statements which, although not necessary parts of the definition itself, indicate circumstances in which the definition does or does not apply.

Diagnose (verb). The process of distinguishing one disease from another.

Diagnosis (noun). The underlying condition or abnormality that is causing the presenting symptoms. In modern scientific medicine, it is often possible to identify an anatomical or biochemical abnormality that is causing the symptoms, that the doctor has learned about during training. A native folk healer (shaman), will give a diagnosis according to the beliefs current in the society of the patient and the healer.

When more than one diagnosis needs to be made, the one requiring the most urgent action, such as treatment or admission, or the one likely to have the most serious consequences in terms of disabilities and prognosis, should be recorded as the **main diagnosis**.

Alternative diagnosis. If a choice has to be made between two possible diagnoses, the most likely should be recorded as the **main diagnosis**, and the other should be recorded as an **alternative diagnosis**, plus a brief narrative comment about the reasons.

Differential diagnosis. When several diagnoses have to be seriously considered, a list of these constitutes the differential diagnosis.

Subsidiary diagnosis. A diagnosis that needs to be made in addition to the main diagnosis, because the patient is suffering from more than one condition. It is not in competition for importance with the main or alternative diagnoses.

Disability. A general umbrella term covering impairments of functions, limitations of activities, and restrictions of participation in social activities (see Appendix 3 on the International Classification of Functions, Disability, and Health: ICF).

Disease. Any known deviation from, or interruption of, the normal structure and function of any part of the body. In the early stages, there may be no obvious effects, but a typical set of symptoms usually develops as the abnormalities progress.

Disease entity. A disease that has an established set of information about its cause, typical symptoms, and possible outcomes.

Disease, illness, and sickness. In ordinary non-medial discourse, these are often used synonymously. But in medical discourse, it is useful to give them separate but related meanings. 'Disease' indicates that there is a known abnormal physical or physiological cause for the symptoms of the patient, 'illness' means the feelings and the experience of the patient, whether or not there is any understandable physical cause for the symptoms, and 'sickness' is the social consequences of the illness. There is further discussion of this important topic in Section 13.1.

Disorder. See sections 13.31,13.32, and 13.33 for slightly different definitions in ICD-10, DSM-IV, and DSM-5.

Entity. A thing that has real existence, demonstrated by its own properties and by known relationships with other entities.

Formulation. In clinical medicine, this is a statement that summarizes the conclusions of whoever is making the statement about the most important aspects of a patient such as causation, clinical state, results of investigations, diagnosis, treatment, and prognosis. It is based upon the **summary** of the unarguable facts about the history and clinical state that are known about the patient. The summary should be the same whoever prepares it, but different clinicians may have different opinions about the relative importance of facts in the summary so that they arrive at different formulations.

Function. In the ICF (see Appendix 3), body functions are defined as 'the physiological functions of body systems (including psychological functions)'. This is little more than a repetition of the word. In a more general sense, any part of the body (including the mind) can be said to be functioning normally when it is doing what other parts of the body need it to do so that they can carry out their own functions.

Glossary. A list of explanations of the meaning of words in a technical document.

Handicap. A hindrance or difficulty that prevents or interferes with the performance of an activity. In the ICIDH (WHO 1980), handicap had a specific but complicated meaning to do with the social consequences of disabilities and impairments. In the now current ICF (WHO 2001a and b) the term handicap is not used.

Hierarchy. An organization of things in grades or levels that are ranked one above the other. Each level in a hierarchy has its own conceptual identity, but also depends upon the level below. Similarly, each level contributes to the concept and functions of the next level above (see chapter note 2 in Chapter 12).

Taxonomic hierarchy. A classification of things that is arranged in a hierarchy of levels. Within each level, there are groups of things with similar characteristics. Each group is a **taxon** (plural: **taxa**).

Impairment. In the ICF (WHO 2001b), impairments are problems in body function or structure due to significant deviation or loss.

Interview. A conversation with a shared purpose or aim, usually between two persons, one of whom takes the lead. Both the interviewer and the interviewee are aware of the purpose of the interview from the start.

Inter-rater reliability. A measure of the degree of agreement between observers when they rate independently the same items of a rating schedule, using the same amount of information (such as both observing an interview, or both reading the same case history).

Lexicon. A dictionary.

Nosology. A branch of medical science dealing with the classification of diseases.

Nosological entity. The same as a disease entity, as noted on p. 115.

Operational definition. A definition of a thing by means of characteristics that can be measured. In psychiatry, this has been extended to include symptoms that can be described with high inter-rater reliability.

Organic causation (organic aetiology). In psychiatry, symptoms may be called **organic** when there is concomitant damage to, or loss of, brain tissue, or interference with physiological brain functions, by a known process. But recent advances in the technology of brain imaging, such as CT, PET, and MRI have shown that there are many instances of definite but minor abnormalities of brain tissue or function that are not accompanied by any detectable symptoms.

The term remains in use for want of anything better.

Pathogenic. Able to cause disease.

Pathoplastic. Able to modify the course or the symptoms of a disease.

Presenting complaint; presenting symptoms. These cause the subject to seek professional help and advice.

Psychosomatic. This term is no longer recommended for use. Previously used to describe physical diseases in which psychological factors were thought to be involved in causation (such as peptic ulcer and asthma).

Repeatability. A measure of agreement when a rating procedure is repeated on a different occasion. For instance, when a subject is interviewed again the next day, by the same rater or by a different rater.

Rubric. Heading of section or chapter, often printed in special lettering or colour.

Standardized interview; structured interview. These terms are often used as equivalents, to mean an interview which is conducted according to a detailed schedule designed to reduce, as much as possible, variation between interviewers in what they ask and what they record. In practice, two varieties of interview have evolved as follows. *Standardized* can be used to indicate that the interviewer asks only questions that are contained in the schedule, following the order in which they are printed, and not asking any other questions or probes (other than repeats). The CIDI and DIS are in this category. *Structured* can be used to indicate that the interviewer follows the main headings and questions in a schedule, but is also free to vary the order of questions, and to ask extra questions so as to clarify obscure replies or obtain additional information that might allow a more definite rating to be made. This covers the PSE and the SCAN.

Signs and symptoms. Physical, physiological, psychological, and behavioural abnormalities which are generally thought by doctors to be indicative of an underlying pathological process. In the physical medicine and surgical disciplines, **symptoms** are often differentiated from signs. **Symptoms** are subjective experiences reported by the patient (such as pain or feelings of anxiety) and **signs** are abnormalities that can be seen or measured objectively (such as physical lumps or deformities). In psychiatry this differentiation is not usually made, and **symptom** is used to cover both.

Syndrome. A group of symptoms that often occur together suggesting that there is an underlying cause, although the exact nature of this is not known. A syndrome also often has a typical time course, response to treatment, and outcome. The best examples in psychiatry are the various types of schizophrenia and depression. As knowledge has progressed in physical medicine, many syndromes have become understandable as diseases, so perhaps the same will occur in the future for psychiatric syndromes.

Taxonomy. The following statements are best regarded as the tip of an iceberg regarding the academic discipline of classification. A conveniently accessible source of more detailed information on this topic is the Wikipedia entry on 'taxonomy': The scientific study or discipline of classification and naming things, particularly living organisms, by means of shared characteristics into groups that indicate natural relationships.

In a **taxonomic hierarchy** things are placed in groups (or **taxon**, plural **taxa**) according to shared characteristics, and each taxon is given a name and placed in a rank or level. If sufficient reliable information is available, the ranks are then ordered to form a 'super group' of higher rank, thus forming a hierarchy of ranks. (see chapter note 2 in Chapter 12).

Validity. (This is a notoriously difficult subject, since several types of validity are recognized.) *In general usage*, this means sound, well defended, legally correct. *In psychological and psychiatric research* it means the extent to which a statement, method, or test, describes or measures what it is supposed to describe or measure. **Validity** and **reliability** are connected in a way not often appreciated (but easy to remember), in that reliability is a measure of the agreement between sets of data about something when the conditions and methods of measurement are *closely similar*, whereas validity is a measure of agreement between different sets of data about something when the conditions and methods of measurement are *widely different* (Anne Anastasi).

Addendum to Section 13.3.3

DSM-5 was published and put on sale in May 2013, just after the text of this book was finalized. However, it is possible to include the definition of disorder used in DSM-5 by the addition of this Addendum.

The definition of mental disorder used in DSM-5

A mental disorder is a syndrome characterized by clinically significant disturbance in an individual's cognition, emotion regulation, or behavior that reflects a dysfunction in the psychological, biological, or developmental processes underlying mental functioning. Mental disorders are usually associated with significant distress or disability in social, occupational, or other important activities. An expectable or culturally approved response to a common stressor or loss, such as the death of a loved one, is not a mental disorder. Socially deviant behavior (e.g. political, religious, or sexual) and conflicts that are primarily between the individual and society are not mental disorders unless the deviance or conflict results from a dysfunction in the individual, as described above.

Comment

The only significant difference in DSM-5 from the definition used in DSM-IV and DSM-IV-TM is the insertion of the word 'usually', i.e. 'Mental disorders are <u>usually</u> associated with significant distress or disability ....etc. (authors' emphasis.)

The wording used in DSM-IV and DSM-IV-TM was 'a clinically significant syndrome or pattern that <u>is</u> associated with present distress or disability .... etc.' (authors' emphasis).

The implications of this change will doubtless be the subject of considerable discussion in the future.

References

Alonso, J., Lépine, J.P., et al. (2007) Overview of key data from the European Study of the Epidemiology of Mental Disorders (ESEMeD). *Journal of Clinical Psychiatry* **68** Suppl 2: 3–9.

Andrews, G., Charney, D.S., Sirovatka, P.J., and Regier, D.A. (Eds) (2009) *Stress-induced and fear circuitry disorders: Refining the research agenda for DSM-V.* American Psychiatric Association, Arlington, Virginia.

Andrews, G., Goldberg, D.P., Krueger, R.F., Carpenter, W.T. jnr., Hyman, S.E., Sachdev, P., Pine, D.S. (2009) Exploring the feasibility of a metastructure for DSM-V and ICD-11: Could it improve utility and validity? *Psychological Medicine* **39**: 1993–2000.

Anthony, J.C, Folstein, M., Romanoski, A.J., et al. (1985) Comparison of lay Diagnostic Interview Schedule and a standardized physcian diagnosis. *Archives of General Psychiatry* **42**: 667–75.

APA (1980a) *Diagnostic and Statistical Manual of Mental Disorders*, Third Edition, APA, Washington DC.

APA (1980b) *Quick Reference to the Diagnostic Criteria from the Diagnostic and Statistical Manual of Mental Disorders*, Third Edition, APA, Washington DC

APA (1994) *Diagnostic and Statistical Manual of Mental Disorders*, Fourth Edition, APA, Washington DC.

APA (2000) *Diagnostic and Statistical Manual of Mental Disorders*, Fourth Edition, Text Revision (DSM-IV-TR) APA, Washington DC.

Baasher, T.A., Cooper, J.E., Davidian, H., et al. (Eds) (1982) Epidemiology and the Mental Health Services: Principles and applications in developing countries. *Acta Psychiatrica Scandinavica* **65** Suppl 285.

Banzato, C.E.M., Rodrigues, A.C.T. (2007) Internationale Psychiatrische Klassifikation: Universalität ohne Essenzialismus. *Die Psychiatrie* **4**: 91–7.

Beach, S.R.H., Wamboldt, M.Z., Kaslow, N.J., Heyman, R.E., First, M.B., Underwood, L.G., and Reiss, D. (Eds) (2006) *Relational processes and DSM-V: Neuroscience, assessment, prevention, and treatment.* APA, Washington DC.

Bebbington, P.E. and Nayani, T. (1995) The Psychosis Screening Questionnaire. *International Journal of Methods in Psychiatric Research* **5**: 11–19.

Berry, J.W. (1969) On cross-cultural comparability. *International Journal of Psychology* **4**: 119–128.

Bickenbach, J.E., Chatterji, S., Badley, E.M., and Ustun, T.B. (1999) Models of disablement, universalism and the ICIDH. *Social Science and Medicine* **48**: 1173–87.

Bilikiewicz, T. (1951) Próba nozograficznego ukladu etioepigenetycznego w psychiatrii. *Neurologia I Neurochirurgia Polska* **13**: 68–78.

Brooke, E.M. (1963) A cohort study of patients first admitted to mental hospitals in 1954 and 1955. *Studies in Medical and Population Subjects No. 18.* HMSO: London.

Brugha, T.S., Jenkins, R., Taub, N., Meltzer, H., and Bebbington, P.E. (2001) A general population comparison of the Composite International Diagnostic Interview (CIDI) and the Schedules for Clinical Assessment in Neuropsychiatry (SCAN). *Psychological Medicine* **31**: 1001–13.

Burke, J.D. jnr (1988) 'Field Trials of the 1987 draft of Chapter V(F) of ICD-10'. In: Psychiatric Classification in an International Perspective. *British Journal of Psychiatry* **152**: Supplement 1 May 1988.

Burvill, P. (1987) An appraisal of the NIMH Epidemiological Catchment Area Program. *Australian and New Zealand Journal of Psychiatry* **21**, No. 2: 175–84

Callard, F., Sartorius, N., Arboledo-Flórez, J., Bartlett, P., Helmchen, H., Stuart, H., Tarboda, J., and Thornicroft, G. (2012) *Mental illness, discrimination, and the Law: Fighting for social justice.* Wiley-Blackwell: Oxford.

Carothers, J.C. (1951) Frontal lobe function and the African. *Journal of Mental Science* **97**: 12–48.

Cooper, J.E. (1967) Diagnostic change in a longitudinal study of psychiatric patients. *British Journal of Psychiatry* **113**: 129–42.

Cooper, J.E, Kendell, R.E, Gurland, B.J., Sartorius, N., and Farkas, T. (1969) Cross-national study of diagnosis of the mental disorders: some results from the first comparative investigation. *American Journal Of Psychiatry* **125**, 10, Supplement: 21–9

Cooper, J.E. (1970) The use of a procedure for standardizing psychiatric diagnosis. In: *Psychiatric Epidemiology: An International Symposium*, E. H. Hare and J. K.Wing (Eds), pages 109–132. Oxford University Press: London.

Cooper, J.E., Kendell, R.E., Gurland, B.J., Sharpe, L., Copeland, J.R.M., and Simon, R. (1972) *Psychiatric Diagnosis in New York and London.* Maudsley Monograph No. 20. Oxford University Press: London.

Cooper, J.E. and Sartorius, N. (1977) Cultural and temporal variations in schizophrenia: A speculation on the importance of industrialization. *British Journal of Psychiatry* **130**: 50–5.

Cooper, J.E. (1982a) Seminars in China. *World Health*, October 1982: 23–5.

Cooper, J.E. (1982b) The last big one? *British Journal of Psychiatry* **141**: 531–2

Cooper, J.E. (1983) Diagnosis and the diagnostic process. In: *Handbook of Psychiatry*, vol 1. Eds M. Shepherd and O.L. Zangwill, Chapter 8, pp 199–209. Cambridge University Press: Cambridge.

Cooper, J.E. (1995) On the publication of the Diagnostic and Statistical Manual of Mental Disorders: Fourth Edition (DSM-IV). *British Journal of Psychiatry* **166**: 4–8.

Cooper, J.E. and Sartorius, N. (1996) (Eds) *Mental Disorders in China.* Gaskell; Royal College of Psychiatrists, London.

Cooper, J.E. (1999) The Classification of Somatoform Disorders in ICD-10. In: *Somatoform Disorders: a Worldwide Perspective*, Y. Ono, A. Janka, M. Asai, N. Sartorius (Eds) *Keio University Symposia for Life Science and Medicine*, vol 3, pages 11–18. Springer Verlag Tokyo.

Dimsdale, J.E., Xin, Yu, Kleinman, A., Patel, V., Narrow, W.E., Sirovatka, P.J., and Regier, D.A. (Eds) (2009) *Somatic presentations of mental disorders: Refining the research agenda for DSM-V.* American Psychiatric Association, Arlington, Virginia.

Eisenberg, L. (1977) Disease and illness: Distinctions between professional and popular ideas of sickness. *Culture, Medicine, and Psychiatry* **1**: 9–23.

Essen-Möller, E. and Wohlfahrt, S. (1947) Suggestions for the amendment of the official Swedish classification of mental disorders. *Acta Psychiatrica Scandinavica* **47** (Suppl): 551–5.

Faris, R.E.L. and Dunham, H.W. (1939) *Mental Illness in Urban Areas.* University Press: Chicago.

Feighner, J.P., Robins, E., Guze, S.B., Woodruff, R. A., Winokur, G., and Munoz, R. (1972) Diagnostic criteria for use in research. *Archives of General Psychiatry* **26**: 57–63.

Ford, C.V. (1983) *The Somatizing Disorders: Illness as a Way of Life.* Elsevier Biomedical: New York, Amsterdam, Oxford.

Fulford, K.W.M. (1989) *Moral theory and medical practice.* Cambridge University Press: Cambridge.

Fulford, W. and Sartorius, N. (2009) The secret history of ICD and the hidden future of DSM. In: *Psychiatry as Cognitive Neuroscience: Philosophical Perspectives*, M. Broome and L. Bortolotti (Eds), pages 29–48. Oxford University Press: Oxford.

Gauron, E.F. and Dickinson, J.K. (1966) Diagnostic decision making in psychiatry. *Archives of General Psychiatry* **14**: 225–37.

Goldberg, E.M. and Morrison, S.L. (1963) Schizophrenia and social class. *British Journal of Psychiatry* **109**: 785–802.

Hamilton, M. (1960) A rating scale for depression. *Journal of Neurology, Neurosurgery, and Psychiatry* **23**(1): 56–62.

Helmchen, H. (1980) Multiaxial systems of classification: Types of axes. *Acta Psychiatrica Scandinavica* **61**: 43–55.

Helzer, J.E., Robins, L.N., McEvoy, L.T., Spitznagel, E.L., Stoltzman, R.K., Farmer, A., and Brockington, I.F (1985) A comparison of clinical and diagnostic interview schedule diagnoses: Physician reexamination of lay-interview cases in the general population. *Archives of General Psychiatry* **42**: 657–66.

Hopper, K., Harrison, G., Janca, A., and Sartorius, N. (2007) Recovery from Schizophrenia: an International Perspective. A report from the WHO Collaborative Project, The International Study of Schizophrenia. Oxford: Oxford University Press.

ICD-10 PHC (1996) Diagnostic and Management Guidelines for Mental Disorders in Primary Care: ICD-10 Chapter V Primary Care Version. WHO/Hogrefe and Huber Publishers: Gottingen, Germany.

Jablensky, A. and Sartorius N., Hirshfeld, R., and Pardes, H. (1983) Diagnosis and classification of mental disorders and alcohol- and drug-related problems: a research agenda for the 1980s. *Psychological Medicine* **13**: 907–21.

Jablensky, A., Sartorius, N., Ernberg, G., Anker, M., Korten, A., Cooper, J.E., Day, R., and Bertelsen, A. (1992) Schizophrenia: manifestations, incidence and course in different cultures: a World Health Organization Ten Country Study. *Psychological Medicine,* Monograph supplement 20

Jablensky, A. (2000) The Epidemiology of Schizophrenia. In: *New Oxford Textbook of Psychiatry,* Eds Gelder, Lopez-Ibor, and Andreasen. Vol 1, Section 4.3.4 pp 585–98.

Jablensky, A. and Kendell, R.E. (2002) Criteria for Assessing a Classification in Psychiatry. In: *Psychiatric Diagnosis and Classification.* Eds: W. Gaebel, J.J. Lopez-Ibor, and N. Sartorius. Chapter 1. Chichester: John Wiley and Sons Ltd.

Jablensky, A. (2012) The disease entity in psychiatry: fact or fiction? *Epidemiology and Psychiatric Sciences* **21**: 265–70.

Jampala, V. S., Sierles F. S., and Taylor M. A. (1986) Consumers' views of DSM-III: Attitudes and practices of US psychiatrists and 1984 graduating psychiatric residents. *American Journal of Psychiatry* **143**: 148–53.

Janca, A., Kastrup, M., Katshnig, H., et al (1996) The ICD-10 multi-axial system for use in adult psychiatry: structure and applications. *Journal of Nervous and Mental Disease* **184**, 191–192.

Karkazis, K. and Feder, E.K. (2008) Naming the problem: disorders and their meanings. *The Lancet* **372**: 2016–7.

Katz, M., Cole, J.O. and Lowery, H.A. (1969) Studies of the diagnostic process: the influence of symptom perception, past experience and ethnic background on diagnostic decisions. *American Journal of Psychiatry* **125**: 937–47.

Kendell, R.E. (1973) Psychiatric diagnoses: a study of how they are made. *British Journal of Psychiatry* **122**: 437–45.

Kendell, R.E. (1975) *The Role of Diagnosis in Psychiatry.* Blackwell Scientific Publications: Oxford, London, Edinburgh.

Kendell, R.E. (1983) The principles of classification in relation to mental disease. In: *Handbook of Psychiatry* vol 1. Eds M. Shepherd and O. L. Zangwill Chapter 7 pp 191–8. Cambridge University Press: Cambridge.

Kendell, R.E., Copeland, J.R.M., Cooper, J.E., Gourlay, J., Sharpe, L. and Gurland, B.J. (1971) *Archives of General Psychiatry* **25**: 123–30

Kessler, R.C., McGonagle, K.A., Zhao, S., Nelson, C.B., Hughes, M., Eshleman, S., Wittchen, H.-U. and Kendler, K.S. (1994) Lifetime and 12-month prevalence of DSM-III-R Psychiatric Disorders in the United States: results from the National Co-morbidity Survey. *Archives of General Psychiatry* **51**(1): 8–19.

Kessler, R.C., Berglund, P., Chiu, W.T., Demler, O., Heeringa, S., Hiripi, E., Jinn, R., Pennel, B-E., Walter, S.D., Zaslavsky, A.M., and Zheng, H. (2004) The US

National Co-Morbidity Survey Replication (NCS-R): an overview of design and field procedures. *International Journal of Methods in Psychiatric Research* **vol 13**, number 2.

Kessler, R.C., Angermeyer, M., Anthony, J.C., De Graaf, R., Demyttennaere, K., et al (2007) Lifetime prevalence and age of onset distributions of mental disorders in the World Health Organization's World Mental Health Survey Initiative. *World Psychiatry* October **6(3)**: 168–76.

Kleinman, A. (1987) Anthropology and Psychiatry: The role of culture in cross-cultural research on illness. *British Journal of Psychiatry* **151**: 447–54.

Kramer, M.(1961) Some problems for international research suggested by observations on differences in first admission rates to the mental hospitals of England and Wales and of the United States. In: *Proceedings of the Third World Congress of Psychiatry* vol 3, pp 153–160. Montreal: University of Toronto Press/ MacGill University Press,

Kramer, M. (1969) Cross-National Study of Diagnosis of the Mental Disorders: Origin of the Problem. *American Journal of Psychiatry* **125.10**: 1–11, Supplement.

Kräupl Taylor, F.K. (1971) A logical analysis of the medico-psychological concept of disease. *Psychological Medicine* **1**: 356–64 and **2**: 7–16.

Kräupl Taylor, F.K. (1976) The medical model of the disease concept. *British Journal of Psychiatry* **128**: 588–94.

Kretschmer, E. (1919) Über psychogenese Wahnbildung bei traumatischer Hirschwäche. *Z Ges Neurol Psychiat*1919 **45**: 272–300.

Kupfer, D.J., First, M.B., and Regier, D.A. (Eds) (2002) A Research Agenda for DSM-V. American Psychiatric Association: Washington D.C.

Leff, J. (1981) *Psychiatry Around the Globe: a trans-cultural view.* Marcel Decker: New York, Basel.

Leme Lopes, J. (1954) *As dimensões do diagnóstico psiquiátrico.* Rio de Janeiro: Agir.

Lewis, A.J. (1934) Melancholia: a clinical survey of depressive states. *Journal of Mental Science,* **80**, 277–378.

Lewis, A.J. (1938) States of Depression: Their Clinical and Aetiological Differentiation. *British Medical Journal* (29 October 1938) **2**: 875–80

Lewis, A.J. (1953) Health as a social concept. *British Journal of Sociology,* **4**: 109–204

Lewis, G., Pelosi, A.J., Araya, R.C., and Dunn, G. (1992) Measuring psychiatric disorder in the community: a standardised assessment for use by lay interviewers. *Psychological Medicine* **22**: 465–86.

Lin, T. (1967) The Epidemiological Study of Mental Disorders. *WHO Chronicle* **21**: 503–16

Lin, T. and Standley, G.C. (1962) The Scope of Epidemiology in Psychiatry. *Public Health Papers No. 16.* World Health Organization: Geneva.

Loranger, A., Sartorius, N., Andreoli, A, Susman, V.L., Oldham, J.L., et al. (1994) The International Personality Disorder Examination (IPDE): the WHO/ ADAMHA international pilot study of personality disorders. *Archives of General Psychiatry* **51**: 215–24.

Maj, M. (2011) Psychiatric Diagnosis: pros and cons of prototypes vs operational criteria. *World Psychiatry*, June **10**(2): 81–2.

Marneros, A. (2004) Die Geburtsstunde der psychiatrischen Wissenschaft und Heilkunde in Deutschland. *Die Psychiatrie* **1**:1–8.

Mellsop, G., Dutu, G., and Robinson, G. (2007) New Zealand psychiatrists views on global features of ICD-10 and DSM-IV. *Australian and New Zealand Journal of Psychiatry* **41**(2):157–65.

Meltzer, H., Gill, B., Petticrew, M., and Hinds, K. (1995) The prevalence of psychiatric morbidity among adults living in private households. *OPCS Surveys of Psychiatric Morbidity in Great Britain. Report 1.* OPCS Social Survey Division. London: HMSO.

Mezzich, J. E. (1979) Patterns and issues in multi-axial psychiatric diagnosis. *Psychological Medicine* **9**: 125–38.

Murphy, H.B. and Raman, A.C. (1971) The chronicity of schizophrenia in indigenous tropical peoples: results of a 12 year follow-up study. *British Journal of Psychiatry* **118**: 489–99

Murphy, J. (1994) The Stirling County Study: then and now. *International Review of Psychiatry* **vol 6 no.4**: 329–48.

Nagi, S.Z. (1965) Some conceptual issues in disability and rehabilitation. In: *Sociology and Rehabilitation* Ed M.B. Sussman pp 110–13. American Sociological Association: Washington DC.

Narrow, W.E., First, M.B., Sirovatka, P.J., and Regier, D.A. (Eds) (2007) *Age and gender considerations in psychiatric diagnosis: A research agenda for DSM-V.* American Psychiatric Association: Arlington, Virginia.

Ottoson, J.O. and Perris, C. (1973) Multidimensional classification of mental disorders. *Psychological Medicine* **3**: 238–43.

Overall, J.E. and Gorham, D.R. (1962) The Brief Psychiatric Rating Scale. *Psychological Reports* **10**: 799–812.

Pareek, U. and Rao, V.(1980) Chapter 2 Cross-cultural surveys and interviewing. In: Triandis, H. C. and Berry J. W. (Eds): *Handbook of Cross-cultural Psychology* Volume 2: Methodology. Boston: Allyn and Bacon.

Parker, G. (1987) (editorial) Are the lifetime prevalence estimates in the ECA study accurate? *Psychological Medicine* **17**: 275–82.

RCPsych (2012) Payment by results for mental health (England). Position Statement PS02/2012, August 2012. Royal College of Psychiatrists: London.

Reed, G.M., Mendonça Correia, J., Esparza, P., Saxena, S., and Maj, M. (2011) The WPA-WHO Global Survey of Psychiatrists' Attitudes Towards Mental Disorders Classifications. *World Psychiatry* **10**: 118–31.

Regier, D.A., Myers, J.K., Kramer, M., Eaton, W.W., Locke, B.Z., Robins, L.N., Blazer, D.G., and Hough, R.L. (1984) The NIMH Epidemiological Catchment Area Programme. *Archives of General Psychiatry* **41**: 934–41.

Regier, D.A., Kaelber, C.T., Roper, M.T., et al. (1994) The ICD-10 clinical field trials for mental and behavioural disorders: results in Canada and the United States. *American Journal of Psychiatry* **151**: 1340–50.

Regier, D.A., Narrow, W.E., Kuhl, E.A., and Kupfer, D.J. (Eds) (2011) *The conceptual evolution of DSM-5*. APA publishing: Washington DC.

Reid, D.D. (1960) *Epidemiological Methods in the study of Mental Disorders*. Health Papers No. 2. Geneva: World Health Organization.

Robins, L.N. and Regier, D.A. (1981) (Eds) *Psychiatric disorders in America: the epidemiological catchment areas study*. Free Press: New York NY.

Robins, L.N., Helzer, J.E., Croughland, J., and Ratcliff, K.S. (1981) National Institute of Mental Health Diagnostic Interview Schedule: its history, characteristics and validity. *Archives of General Psychiatry* **41**: 281–9.

Robins, L.N., Helzer, J.E., Ratcliff, K.S., and Seyfried, W. (1982) Validity of the Diagnostic Interview Schedule Version II: DSM-III Diagnoses. *Psychological Medicine* **12**: 555–70.

Robins, L.N., Helzer, J.E., et al. (1984) Lifetime prevalence of specific psychiatric disorders in three sites. *Archives of General Psychiatry* **41**: 949–58.

Robins, L.N., Wing, J., Wittchen, H.-U., Helzer, J.E., Babor, T.F., Burke, J., Farmer, A., Jablensky, A., Pickens, R., Regier, D.A., et al. (1988) The Composite International Diagnostic Interview. An epidemiologic instrument suitable for use in conjunction with different diagnostic systems and in different cultures. *Archives of General Psychiatry* Dec **45**(12): 1069–77.

Rutter, M., Lebovici, S., Eisenberg, L., et al. (1969) A tri-axial classification of mental disorders in childhood. *Journal of Child Psychology and Psychiatry* **10**: 41–61.

Rutter, M., Schaffer, D., and Shepherd, M. (1975) *A Multi-Axial Classification of Child Psychiatric Disorders*. Geneva: World Psychiatric Organization.

Sandifer, M.G., Horden, A., Timbury, G.C., and Green, M. (1968) Psychiatric Diagnosis: a comparative study in North Carolina, London, and Glasgow. *British Journal of Psychiatry* **114**: 1–9.

Sandifer, M.G., Hordern, A., and Green, L.M. (1970) The Psychiatric Interview: the impact of the first three minutes. *American Journal of Psychiatry* **126**: 968–73.

Sartorius, N. (1973) Culture and the Epidemiology of Depression *Psychiatrica Neurologia Neurochirigia* **76**: 479–87.

Sartorius, N. (1976) Classification: an international perspective. *Psychiatry Annual* **6**: 22–35.

Sartorius, N. (1988) International perspectives of psychiatric classification. In: 'Psychiatric classification in an international perspective', *The British Journal of Psychiatry* **152**, Supplement 1: 9–14.

Sartorius, N., Jablensky, A., Cooper, J.E., and Burke, J.D. (1988) Supplement 1, *British Journal of Psychiatry* **152**: May 1988.

Sartorius, N., Jablensky, A., Regier, D.A., Burke, J.D., and Hirschfeld, R.M.A. (1990) Eds *Sources and Traditions of Classification in Psychiatry*. Hogrefe and Huber: Toronto, Gottingen.

Sartorius, N. (1995) *Understanding the ICD-10 Classification of Mental Disorders*. London: Science Press.

Sartorius, N. (2002) *The Mental Health Adventure of the World Health Organization*. In: *Fighting for Mental Health*. Cambridge University Press: Cambridge UK.

Sartorius, N. and Schulze, H. (2005) *Reducing the Stigma of Mental Illness.* Cambridge University Press: Cambridge UK.

Sartorius, N. (2011) Meta effects of classifying mental disorders. In: *The Conceptual Evolution of DSM 5* (Eds D.A. Regier, W.E. Narrow, E.A. Kuhl and D. Kupfer), pp. 59–80. American Psychiatric Publishing: Arlington, VA.

Sato, M. (2006) Renaming schizophrenia: a Japanese perspective. *World Psychiatry* 5: 53–5.

Saxena, S., Esparza, P., Regier, D.A., Saraceno, B., and Sartorius, N. (Eds) (2012) Public health aspects of diagnosis and classification of mental and behavioral disorders: Refining the research agenda for DSM-5 and ICD-11. American Psychiatric Association, Arlington, Virginia and World Health Organization, Geneva, Switzerland.

Scadding, J.G. (1967) Diagnosis, the clinician, and the computer. *The Lancet (ii):* 877–82.

Schneider, F. (2011) Statement of the President of the German Association for Psychiatry and Psychotherapy. In: *Psychiatry under National Socialism.* Springer Verlag: Heidelberg.

Shepherd, M., Brooke, E.M., Cooper, J.E., and Lin, T. (1968) An Experimental Approach to Psychiatric Diagnosis: an International Study. *Acta Psychiatrica Scandinavica;* Supplement 201.

Simon, G.E., Katon, W.J., and Sparks, B.J. (1990) Allergic to life: psychological factors in environmental illness. *American Journal of Psychiatry* **147**: 1001–6.

Skodol, A.E. (1987) Education and training. In: *An annotated bibliography of DSM-III.* (Eds A. Skodol and R.L. Spitzer) Washington: American Psychiatric Press.

Spitzer, R.L., Fleiss, J., Burdock, E.I., and Hardesty, A.S. (1964) The Mental Status Schedule: rationale, reliability, and validity. *Comprehensive Psychiatry* 5: 384–95.

Spitzer, R.L. and Endicott, J. (1968) DIAGNO: A computer program for psychiatric diagnosis utilizing the differential diagnostic procedure. *Archives of General Psychiatry* **18**: 746–56.

Spitzer, R.L., Endicott, J., Fleiss, J. L., and Cohen, J. (1970) The Psychiatric Status Schedule: a technique for evaluating psychopathology and impairment in role functioning. *Archives of General Psychiatry* **23**: 41–5.

Spitzer, R.L., Endicott, J., and Robins, E. (1975) *Research Diagnostic Criteria for a selected group of functional disorders.* New York State Department of Mental Hygiene, Biometrics Branch.

Srole, L., Lagner, T. S., Michael, S.T., Opler, M.K., and Rennie, T.A.C. (1962) *The Mid-town Manhattan Study: Mental Health in the Metropolis.* McGraw-Hill: New York, Toronto, London.

Stengel, E. (1960) Classification of Mental Disorders. *Bulletin of the World Health Organization* **21**: 601–63.

Sunderland, T., Jeste, D.V., Baiyewu, O., Sirovatka, P.J., and Regier, D.A. (Eds) (2007) *Diagnostic issues in dementia: advancing the research agenda for DSM-V.* American Psychiatric Association: Arlington, Virginia.

Ustun, T.B. and Sartorius N. (1995) (Eds) *Mental Illness in General Health Care: an International Study.* John Wiley and Sons Ltd: Chichester; New York; Toronto.

Van Voren, R. (2010) Abuse of psychiatry for political purposes in the USSR: a case study and personal account of the efforts to bring them to an end. In: Helmchen, H. and Sartorius, N. (Eds) (2010) 'Ethics in Psychiatry—European contributions'. *International Library of Ethics, Law, and the New Medicine* **45**: 489–508. Springer Dordrecht: Heidelberg, London, New York.

von Cranach, M. and Schneider, F. (2010) *In Memoriam: Remembrance and responsibility (Exhibition catalogue)* Springer Verlag: Berlin.

Westen, D. (2012) Prototype diagnosis of psychiatric syndromes. In: Forum: Advantages and Disadvantages of a Prototype-matching Approach to Psychiatric Diagnosis. *World Psychiatry* **11**, number 1: 16–21.

WHO (1966) *Multi-Axial Classification of Child and Adolescent Psychiatric Disorders.* Cambridge: Cambridge University Press.

WHO (1967) *International Classification of Diseases*, 8th Revision. Geneva: World Health Organization.

WHO (1974) *Glossary of Mental Disorders and Guide to their Classification: for use in conjunction with the International Classification of Diseases*, 8th Revision. Geneva: World Health Organization.

WHO (1975) Schizophrenia: a Multinational Study. Public Health Papers 63. Geneva: World Health Organization.

WHO (1980) *International Classification of Impairments, Disabilities, and Handicaps (ICIDH): A manual of classification relating to the consequences of disease.* Geneva: World Health Organization.

WHO (1992) A tri-axial classification of health problems encountered in Primary Health Care; a WHO multi-centre study. Clare A., Gulbinat W., Sartorius N., *Social Psychiatry and Epidemiology* **27**: 108–116.

WHO (1992a) *Mental Health Programmes: Concepts and Principles.* Geneva: Division of Mental Health. World Health Organization (Document WHO/MNH/92.11)

WHO (1992b): *The ICD-10 Classification of Mental and Behavioural Disorders: Clinical Descriptions and Diagnostic Guidelines.* Geneva: World Health Organization.

WHO (1993) *The ICD-10 Classification of Mental and Behavioural Disorders: Diagnostic Criteria for Research (DCR-10).* Geneva: World Health Organization.

WHO (1996) *ICD-10 PHC: Diagnostic and Management Guidelines for Mental Disorders in Primary care.* ICD-10 Chapter V Primary Care Version. Hogrefe and Huber/WHO: Seattle, Toronto, Bern, Gottingen.

WHO (1997) *Multi-Axial presentation of the ICD-10 for Use in Adult Psychiatry.* Cambridge: Cambridge University Press.

WHO (2001a) *International Classification of Functioning, Disability and Health (ICF).* Geneva: World Health Organization.

WHO (2001b) *International Classification of Functioning, Disability and Health (ICF) Short version.* Geneva: World Health Organization.

Wing, J.K., Birley, J.T.L., Cooper, J.E., Graham, P., and Isaacs, A. (1967) Reliability of a procedure for measuring and classifying 'present mental state'. *British Journal of Psychiatry* **113**: 499–515.

Wing, J.K., Cooper, J.E., and Sartorius, N. (1974) *The Measurement and Classification of Psychiatric Symptoms.* Cambridge University Press: Cambridge, London, New York.

Wing, J.K., Babor, T., Brugha, T., Burke, J.D., Cooper, J.E., Giel, R., Jablensky, A., Regier, D., and Sartorius, N. (1990) SCAN: Schedule for Clinical Assessment in Neuropsychiatry. *Archives of General Psychiatry* **47**: 499–515.

Wing, J.K., Sartorius, N., and Ustun, B. (1998) *Diagnosis and clinical measurement in psychiatry: A reference manual for SCAN*, pp. 44–58, Cambridge University press: Cambridge.

Wonca (1986) IC-Process-PC (International Classification of Process in Primary Care). Prepared by the Classification Committee of WONCA (World Organization of National Colleges, Academies, and Academic Associations of General Practitioners/Family Physicians) in collaboration with the Classification Committee of NAPCRG (North American Primary Care Research Group). Oxford University Press: Oxford, New York, Tokyo (2004). International Classification of Primary Care Version 2 (Print on demand).

Wooton, B. (1959) Social pathology and the concepts of mental health and mental illness. In: *Social science and social pathology*. Allen and Unwin: London.

Zimmerman, M. and Gallione, J. (2010) Psychiatrists' and Nonpsychiatrist Physicians' Reported Use of the DSM-IV Criteria for Major Depressive Disorder. *Journal of Clinical Psychiatry* **71 (3):** 235–8.

Zubin, J. (1969) Cross-national study of diagnoses of the mental disorders: methodology and planning *American Journal of Psychiatry* **125** (April 1969 Supplement): 12–20.

Other useful references

Cooper, J.E. (1994) Notes on unsolved problems. In: *Pocket guide to the ICD-10 classification of mental and behavioural disorders (ICD-10 :DCR-10)* pages 345–54. Churchill Livingstone/ Elsevier: Edinburgh, London, New York.

Sartorius, N. and Janca, A. (1996) Psychiatric instruments developed by the World Health Organization. *Social Psychiatry and Psychiatric Epidemiology* **31**: 55–69.

Sartorius, N., Janca, A., Saxena, S., and Üstün, B. (2010) Psychiatric assessment instruments developed by the World Health Organization. In: Thornicroft, G., Tansella, M. (Eds). *Mental Health Outcome Measures* (third edition). London: Royal College of Psychiatrists: p. 281–312.

Tansella, M. (2010) (Ed.). *Mental Health Outcome Measures* (third edition). London: Royal College of Psychiatrists: pp. 281–312.

WHO (1994) ICD-10 Symptom glossary for mental disorders: a glossary of symptoms used in the definition of criteria for the classification of mental and behavioural disorders. In: *The 10th Revision of the International Classification of Diseases (ICD-10)*. WHO: Geneva. Prepared by Isaac, M., Janca, A., and Sartorius, N.

Author index

Subject index

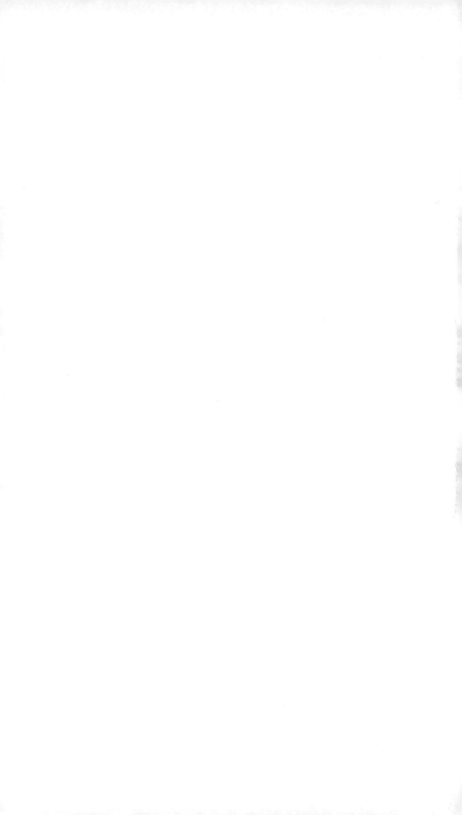